PROTEIN BIOCHEMISTRY, SYNTHESIS, STRUCTURE AND CELLULAR FUNCTIONS

APOLIPOPROTEINS

REGULATORY FUNCTIONS, HEALTH EFFECTS AND ROLE IN DISEASE

Protein Biochemistry, Synthesis, Structure and Cellular Functions

Additional books in this series can be found on Nova's website
under the Series tab.

Additional e-books in this series can be found on Nova's website
under the e-book tab.

Protein Science and Engineering

Additional books in this series can be found on Nova's website
under the Series tab.

Additional e-books in this series can be found on Nova's website
under the e-book tab.

PROTEIN BIOCHEMISTRY, SYNTHESIS, STRUCTURE AND CELLULAR FUNCTIONS

APOLIPOPROTEINS

REGULATORY FUNCTIONS, HEALTH EFFECTS AND ROLE IN DISEASE

ADRIK D. SIDOROV
AND
MISHA Y. NIKITIN
EDITORS

NOVA BIOMEDICAL
New York

For permission to use material from this book please contact us:
Telephone 631-231-7269; Fax 631-231-8175
Web Site: http://www.novapublishers.com

Additional color graphics may be available in the e-book version of this book.

Library of Congress Cataloging-in-Publication Data

ISBN: 978-1-62257-484-1

Library of Congress Control Number: 2012942456

Published by Nova Science Publishers, Inc. † New York

Contents

Preface

Apolipoproteins are proteins that bind lipids (oil-soluble substances such as fat and cholesterol) to form lipoproteins. They transport the lipids through the lymphatic and circulatory systems. Apolipoproteins also serve as enzyme cofactors, receptor ligands, and lipid transfer carriers that regulate the metabolism of lipoproteins and their uptake in tissues. In this book, the authors present current research in the study of the regulatory functions, health effects and role in disease of apolipoproteins. Topics include macrophages, apolipoproteins, steroid hormones and molecular mechanisms of cell proliferation; formation of discoidal apolipoprotein A-1 lipid bound complexes; the role of apolipoprotein E in cardiovascular and renal disease; the functional variants and mutations of the apolipoprotein A5 gene in human pathology; and regulation of FGF-1 of ApoE/HDL generation in astrocytes.

Chapter I - At hepatectomized rats it was shown that immediately after partial liver removal (PLR) the Kupffer macrophages were accumulated in liver remnant. At the maximal mitotic activity (36 hours following PLR) the relative amount of Kupffer cells keeps low, but 72 hours later turns out to be higher again. The periodic changes of the Kupffer cell amount in hepatectomized rats are accompanied by remarkable increase (1.5 - 3 fold) of free and total lysosomal enzyme activity (acid DNA-ase, acid RNA-ase, cathepsin D). The activation of the Kupffer macrophage lysosomes goes ahead of labilization of hepatocyte lysosomal membranes. The blockade of mononuclear phagocyte system by means of carbonate iron overloading in the early prereplicative period leads to an as long as 10 – 12 hours retardation of hepatocyte proliferation. Kupffer cell activation by means of intravenous injection of bacterial lipopolysaccharides shifted of mitotic activity to the 24 hours after the operation.

Participation of macrophages in molecular mechanisms of cell proliferation is connected with formation of tetrahydrocortisol – apolipoprotein A-I complex. This complex specifically interacts with DNA of hepatocytes rat. In the process of interaction, rupture of hydrogen bonds between the pairs of nitrous bases occurs with the formation of single-stranded DNA structures. In such state DNA forms complexes with DNA polymerase. The most probable site of binding the tetrahydrocortisol – apolipoprotein A-I complex with DNA is the sequence of $CC(GCC)_n$ type entering the structure of many genes, among them the structure of human apolipoprotein A-I gene. Oligonucleotide of this type has been synthesized. Association constant (K_{ass}) of it with tetrahydrocortisol – apolipoprotein A-I complex was shown to be $1.66 \cdot 10^6$ M^{-1}. Substitution of tetrahydrocortisol for cortisol in the complex results in a considerable decrease of K_{ass}. It was assumed that in the GC-pairs of the given sequence tetrahydrocortisol itself participates in the formation of hydrogen bonds with cytosine, favoring their rupture with complementary base – guanine. This mechanism is the basis of DNA replication during cell division.

Chapter II - The double belt model for lipid-bound discoidal apolipoprotein A-I consists of two alpha-helical monomers bound about an unilamellar bilayer of lipids. Previous work, based on salt bridge calculations, has demonstrated that the L5/5 registration, Milano mutant, and Paris mutant are preferred conformations for apolipoprotein A-I. Additional recent research has indicated that there is a possibility of inter-ring rotation between the two monomers about the lipid unilamellar bilayer core. For instance, from well-known mutations, the Paris (R151C) and Milano (R173C) mutants indicate a mode of change must be available. To find proper registration, one proposed change is a 'rotationally' independent circular motion of the two protein monomers about the lipid unilamellar bilayer core. Current research shows that from a computational perspective, the independent inter-ring rotation of the two alpha-helical monomers about the lipid unilamellar bilayer core is feasible. And, such simulations support the existing double-belt model. Other long time scale dynamics simulations are very revealing of the discoidal behavior having preferred out-of-plane shapes akin to a saddle-point. However, despite all of the indicated deformations, the rotation of the two protein monomers is able to occur with biasing. It was determined that a cysteine mutant at Glu107 as a possible target for future mutational studies. Several other biophysical studies are discussed in light of these recent findings to bring a greater understanding to ApoA-I dynamic motion and registration shifts. Since HDL remodeling is necessary for cholesterol transport, our model for remodeling through dynamics has substantial biomedical implications.

Chapter III - It is well established that apolipoproteins play a crucial role in serum lipids transport and metabolism. Particularly, the apolipoprotein E (apoE) is mainly involved in the transport of very-low density lipoproteins and intermediary density lipoproteins by the liver, but new insights revealed a wide range of functions performed by apoE. This lipoprotein is related to the modulation of inflammatory process and regulates the expression of multiple genes in various diseases. Besides, apoE isoforms are involved in progression of cardiovascular and renal diseases. This chapter presents a review about the achievements in both experimental and clinical studies that contribute to understanding the role of apoE in both physiological and pathological situations. Focus now is on the participation of apoE as a key modulatory factor to the development of atherosclerosis, diabetes and kidney diseases and the contributions of available animal models to clarify the mechanisms involved in these pathologies in humans.

Chapter IV - One of the many factors affecting the lipid metabolism by a complex manner is the apolipoprotein A-5 (ApoA5). The gene of the *ApoA5* is located on chromosome 11q23 in the *ApoA1/C3/A4/A5* gene cluster. With a moderate rage of circulating plasma ApoA5 concentration (50-250 ng/ml), it plays an effective regulatory role in triglyceride metabolism. In the plasma, the protein is found mainly on TG rich lipoproteins such as chylomicrons and VLDL where it shows an opposite effect as the ApoC3, namely enhancing lipoprotein lipase mediated triglyceride catabolism. It comes from this key role of the ApoA5, that the common naturally occurring variants (like T-1131C, T1259C, C56G, and IVS3+G476A) and haplotypes determined by them are associated with elevated plasma triglyceride concentrations, these variants and haplotype combinations have been shown to confer risk or protection for development of cardiovascular disease, stroke and metabolic syndrome. However, there are also some less frequent genetic variants that in combination with the common allelic variants of the gene can define haplotypes that are associated with more pronounced triglyceride level increase. In addition, there are rare mutations of the *ApoA5* gene which are associated with specific complex phenotype that includes extremely high triglyceride levels with multiple organ pathology. The current chapter summarizes these three groups represented by point mutations, deletion/insertion mutations, splicing mutations, and associate with different human pathology.

Chapter V - It is known that lipoproteins and lipopolysaccharide binding protein bind lipopolysaccharide in blood plasma and play important role in the mechanism of anti-inflammatory protection. The aim of the present study was to investigate the role of high-density lipoproteins and apolipoprotein A-I in binding, transport and neutralization of bacterial lipopolysaccharide. The authors used the high-density lipoproteins (HDL), apolipoprotein A-I (apoA-I), rat hepatocytes, tumor-associated macrophages (TAMs), and lipopolysaccharide (LPS) from Escherichia coli. To study interactions of LPS and HDL tryptophan fluorescence quenching and electrophoretic mobilities in agarose gel is used. Results suggest a physical interaction of HDL with LPS. ApoA-I, the main protein component of HDL, plays a crucial role in LPS binding to HDL. Pathological effect of LPS is mediated by proinflammatory cytokines secreted by macrophages. The increased secretion of some cytokines is harmful for neighboring cells. For example, the ability of IL-1β to increase metastatic potential of a tumor is well known. It is considered that interaction of HDL with LPS prevent the activation of macrophages. Also, the treatment of TAMs culture with LPS-HDL complexes decreased an intracellular IL-1β concentration in TAMs. The effect of HDL may be caused by participation of apoA-I in regulation of expression of genes of proinflammatory cytokines in macrophages or with endocytosis of LPS with HDL through macrophages HDL-receptors, without participation Toll-like receptor and activation of cytokine genes. Using the fluorescent microscopy and spectrofluorimetry we found the ability of apoA-I to carry fluorescein isothiocyanate labeled LPS into rat hepatocytes. It is known, that LPS does not interact directly with hepatocytes. The authors suppose that complex LPS with apoA-I interacts with a HDL-receptor and gets into cells by endocytosis and then can be exposed to metabolic degradation in hepatocytes. Our date indicates that hepatocytes take place in LPS clearance as a complex with HDL bypassing macrophages. Neutralization of LPS by HDL can be considered as alternative and safe way, allowing to prevent an activation of macrophages and decreases the inflammatory response. The results of the present study demonstrate that HDL and apoA-I may play an important role in LPS binding and prevent acute inflammatory response and development of metabolic diseases.

Chapter VI - Major output of the numerous studies of LCAT activity toward HDL with apoA-I is restricted by only two and bulk values. Moreover, the contributions of LCAT binding to HDL surface and apoA-I structure to LCAT action at interface have not been evaluated. In the present study cholesterol is considered as alcoholic nucleophile that increases the solvolysis rate of acyl-LCAT intermediate. A complete set of individual rate constants for the formation of acyl-enzyme intermediate (k_2), its hydrolysis/solvolysis by water (k_3) and cholesterol (k_4) may be derived from a full kinetic equation that describes the interface velocity in terms of the initial surface concentrations of phosphatidylcholine and cholesterol in discoidal HDL. This analysis was applied to discover the contribution of 139-170 central region of apoA-I molecule to LCAT activation by apolipoprotein. LCAT binding to individual preparations of HDL with Δ139-170 apoA-I deletion mutant or plasma apoA-I was measured with a solid phase assay. The raw kinetic data of Holvoet et al. (Biochemistry (1995) 34: 13334-13342) for these HDL preparations were fitted also with model dependencies of on k_4 within wide range of k_2 and k_3 values. The 139-170 region in apoA-I sequence influences mainly the proper positioning of cholesterol molecule toward LCAT active center, local arginine residue(s) is suggested to contribute primarily. The analysis may be extended for other apoA-I mutations affecting LCAT activity.

Chapter VII - The neural cells in the central nervous system (CNS) are segregated by the blood-brain barrier (BBB) from cholesterol transporters such as low density lipoproteins (LDL) and very low density lipoproteins (VLDL) in human blood plasma, although the CNS is an organ to require cholesterol at very high level. Therefore, cholesterol homeostasis in the CNS is surely controlled by the brain-specific cholesterol transport system. Apolipoprotein E (apoE) produced by astrocytes is a most abundant apolipoprotein in the cerebrospinal fluid (CSF). Astrocytes generate cholesterol-rich high density lipoprotein (apoE/HDL) by using the endogenous apoE and phospholipid-rich and cholesterol-poor HDL (apoA-I/HDL) through the interaction with exogenous apoA-I which is probably produced by brain endothelial cells.

The secretion of endogenous apoE from rat astrocytes is started within 30 min after the initiation of biosynthesis. The apoE secreted from rat astrocytes uses pre-synthesized cholesterol rather than newly-synthesized cholesterol for biogenesis of HDL, although exogenous human apoE mediates effluxes of both pre-synthesized and newly synthesized cholesterols as well as exogenous cyclodextrin. This suggests that astrocytes secrete hardly endogenous apoE as a lipid-free apoE.

Rat astrocytes cultured for one month (long-term cultured astrocytes) enhance significantly generation of apoE/HDL dependently on fibroblast growth factor 1 (FGF-1) produced by astrocytes in the manner of apparent autocrine action. The release of FGF-1 is likely provoked by oxidative stress involved in long-term cultured stress. Purified FGF-1 enhances the apoE/HDL generation of astrocytes accompanied with enhancing syntheses of both apoE and cholesterol. FGF-1 increases cholesterol synthesis through the activation of MAP kinase cascade in astrocytes, stimulates intracellular apoE transport through PI3-kinase/Akt pathway and enhances apoE mRNA expression through increasing mRNA expression of LXRα.

The mechanism underlying FGF-1 release from astrocytes and subsequent generation of apoE/HDL are important issues to be addressed to understand the role of FGF-1 in damaged brains, including bran injury, brain inflammation, or neurodegenerative diseases. The regulation by FGF-1 of apoE/HDL generation under the stress-conditions is mainly argued on the base of our experimental results including recently obtained and unpublished several data in this chapter.

In: Apolipoproteins
Editors: A. D. Sidorov and M. Y. Nikitin
ISBN: 978-1-62257-484-1

Chapter I

Macrophages, Lipo (APO) Proteins, Steroid Hormones, and Molecular Mechanisms of Cell Proliferation

L. E. Panin
Scientific Research Institute of Biochemistry SB RAMS,
Novosibirsk, Russia

Abstract

At hepatectomized rats it was shown that immediately after partial liver removal (PLR) the Kupffer macrophages were accumulated in liver remnant. At the maximal mitotic activity (36 hours following PLR) the relative amount of Kupffer cells keeps low, but 72 hours later turns out to be higher again. The periodic changes of the Kupffer cell amount in hepatectomized rats are accompanied by remarkable increase (1.5 - 3 fold) of free and total lysosomal enzyme activity (acid DNA-ase, acid RNA-ase, cathepsin D). The activation of the Kupffer macrophage lysosomes goes ahead of labilization of hepatocyte lysosomal membranes. The blockade of mononuclear phagocyte system by means of carbonate iron overloading in the early prereplicative period leads to an as long as 10 – 12 hours retardation of hepatocyte proliferation. Kupffer cell activation by means of intravenous injection of bacterial lipopolysaccharides shifted of mitotic activity to the 24 hours after the operation.

Participation of macrophages in molecular mechanisms of cell proliferation is connected with formation of tetrahydrocortisol – apolipoprotein A-I complex. This complex specifically interacts with DNA of hepatocytes rat. In the process of interaction, rupture of hydrogen bonds between the pairs of nitrous bases occurs with the formation of single-stranded DNA structures. In such state DNA forms complexes with DNA polymerase. The most probable site of binding the tetrahydrocortisol – apolipoprotein A-I complex with DNA is the sequence of $CC(GCC)_n$ type entering the structure of many genes, among them the structure of human apolipoprotein A-I gene. Oligonucleotide of this type has been synthesized. Association constant (K_{ass}) of it with tetrahydrocortisol – apolipoprotein A-I complex was shown to be $1.66 \cdot 10^6$ M^{-1}. Substitution of tetrahydro-cortisol for cortisol in the complex results in a considerable decrease of K_{ass}. It was assumed that in the GC-pairs of the given sequence tetrahydrocortisol itself participates in the formation of hydrogen bonds with cytosine, favoring their rupture with complementary base – guanine. This mechanism is the basis of DNA replication during cell division.

1. Introduction

Molecular mechanisms of cell proliferation are of great interest not only in terms of physiological regulation of organs and tissues regeneration, but also in terms of possible tumor growth. These mechanisms are commonly investigated using chemical tissue damage (CCL_4 hepatitis) and partial liver resection (PLR) as models [1, 2]. The latter model is most interesting for studying the regulatory mechanisms of regeneration. It was shown that enhancement of protein biosynthesis, including transcription and growth factors as well as signal transmitting proteins, starts within 5-6 h after partial hepatectomy (G1 phase) [3]. Enhancement of DNA synthesis (S phase) is observed 10-12 h after the surgery. Its maximum in hepatocytes corresponds to 36 h; in Kupffer and stellate cells, to 48 h; and in endotheliocytes of hepatic sinusoids, to 96 h. Transitions between phases of the cell cycle depends on the interaction of cyclins, cyclin-dependent kinases and their inhibitors [4, 5, 6]. The entire regeneration process terminates in 7-10 days [7].

The priming phase is characterized by the expression of immediate early genes. It increases the activity of such transcription factors as NF kappa B, STAT3, AP-1, AP-2, GATA, PAX-6, C/EBP alpha and beta, and others. This is followed by a phase at which the expression of cell cycle genes is enhanced. It increases the activity of growth factors, in particular, hepatocyte (HGF), transforming (TGF-α), epidermal (EGF), vascular endothelial (VEGF), basic fibroblast (BFGF), insulin-like growth factors (IGF) 1 and 2, etc. [4, 8, 9]. HGF, interacting with other growth factors, is essential for stimulation of DNA synthesis in hepatocytes [10].

The mechanism of DNA synthesis enhancement is strongly contributed by glucocorticoids (cortisol and corticosterone) [10]. It was shown that small doses of cortisol facilitate proliferation of hepatocytes, whereas large doses suppress it [11]. The role of cortisol is related not only to enhancing the DNA synthesis, but also to raising the activity of histone-associated proteinase [12]. The enhancement of nucleolar RNA synthesis was noted earlier [13]. Later these mechanisms were thoroughly studied in our works. It was revealed that the active form of cortisol, which enhances gene expression, is represented by its reduced species — tetrahydrocortisol (THC) [14], whereas apolipoprotein A-I (apoA-I) serves as a transport form transferring the hormone to hepatocyte nuclei [15]. ApoA-I is the major constituent of high density lipoproteins (HDL_3). In liver regeneration, lipoproteins (LP) serve also as a source of vitamin E (antioxidants) [16], signal phospholipids (phosphatidylinositols and sphingomyelins) [17], and certainly as a source of building material (cholesterol and phospholipids) necessary for the formation of biological membranes [18]. A great contribution to regeneration mechanisms is made by the metabolic relations of macrophages and hepatocytes.

On these grounds, we investigated the role of macrophages, cortisol, and serum lipoproteins in biosynthesis of apolipoproteins, protein, DNA, and other mechanisms affecting cell proliferation after partial liver resection.

2. Material and Methods

2.1. The Model of Investigation

Sixty male Wistar strain rats weighting 180-200 g were hepatectomized by Higgins and Anderson method [19]. In each case 2/3 of total liver mass was removed. Five to seven rats were sacrificed by decapitation at 2, 5, 9, 24, 36 and 72 hours after partial liver resection (PLR). In control series the specimens of liver from sham-operated rats were employed. The liver tissue was fixed in buffered formaldehyde or Carnoy mixture, the slices were stained with hematoxyline-eosine and Shiff-reagent according to Feulgen method. In 5 mcm thick liver slices the relative number of mitoses per 8000 hepatocytes and the amount of Kupffer cells per 1000 hepatocytes were determined.

In special experiments the liver regeneration was studied under the overloading of Kupffer cells with colloid iron particles. The Kupffer cell blockade has been performed 2 hours before or 3 and 18 hours after PLR. For this aim rats received through v. femoralis injections of 2 ml of 5% carbonyl-phosphate colloid iron (type R-100F, particle size 0.8-1.5 mcm) suspended in isotonic 5% starch solution. Kupffer cell activation has been performed by intravenous injection of bacterial lipopolysaccharides (LPS) isolated from Serratia marcescens (0.25 mg/kg).

2.2. Biochemical Methods

The enzyme activities were determined in whole liver homogenates as well as in hepatocytes and Kupffer cell fractions. The total and free (in presence of 0.1% Triton X-100) acid DNA-ase, acid RNA-ase [20] and cathepsin D [21] were estimated. The total protein content was assayed according to Lowry [22]. 11-oxycorticosteroids in blood serum were determined fluorometrically [23]. The total fraction of LDL and VLDL in blood serum and in supernatant fraction of liver homogenate was found by heparin precipitation in the presence of $CaCl_2$. Electrophoresis of blood serum lipoproteins was performed according to Lammley [24]. The rate of protein synthesis in organs and tissues was determined in vivo from ^{14}C-leucine incorporation. For this purpose, the animals were intraperitoneally injected with labeled leucine at a dose of 25 μCi per 100 g of body weight 2 h before slaughter. The rate of DNA synthesis in organs and tissues was estimated from incorporation of ^{3}H-thymidine into DNA. This was made by intraperitoneal injection of ^{3}H-thymidine at a dose of 10 μCi per 100 g of body weight 1 h before slaughter .

Radioactivity of DNA and of total protein was measured by β-counter 'Multimat-30' (France). For radioactivity determination of DNA, homogenate aliquots were placed to GF/C filters, which were six times washed by 5 ml of cooled 10% trichloracetic acid (TCA), and then by 5 ml of 95% ethanol. For radioactivity determination of proteins, homogenate aliquotes were placed at FN-16 filters pretreated by 0.1 M leucine solution in 10% TCA. The filters were subsequently washed in TCA solution and ethanol-ether. Specific radioactivity was calculated for 1 mg of a protein measured by the method of Lowry.

2.3. Analysis of HDL and Cortisol Effects on Chromatin Activity in the Liver Cell Nuclei

Cell nuclei were isolated from surviving rat liver sections incubated with HDL (0.2 mg/ml of the medium) and cortisol ($3{\cdot}10^{-6}$ M). Intracellular transport was suppressed by vinblastin (10^{-6} M) and colchicine ($5{\cdot}10^{-7}$ M). Pepstatin, iodoacetamide, and soybean inhibitor of trypsin were used to inhibit the activity of lysosomal enzymes. The obtained nuclei were resuspended in a 0.05 M citrate-phosphate buffer with pH 4.4, which contained 0.15 M NaCl and 2 mM $MgCl_2$, and incubated with acridine orange (AO) for 30 min. Fluorescence was measured on a MPF-4 Hitachi (Japan) spectrofluorimeter. The number of binding sites was calculated according to [26].

2.4. Preparation of the Fraction of Acidic Nonhistone Proteins of the Nuclei Isolated from Various Tissues

To remove histone proteins, the nuclei were homogenized for 2 min in a solution of 0.075 M NaCl and 0.025 M EDTA Na_2 at pH 7.5 and centrifuged for 30 min at 2000 g. The sediment was homogenized for 1 min in the initial NaCl/EDTA solution and centrifuged for 30 min at 2000 g. The sediment was washed twice in the same solution, each time for 30 s, with subsequent centrifuging for 15 min at 2000 g. Acidic nonhistone proteins were extracted three times using a 0.35 M solution of NaCl. The obtained sediment was homogenized for 1 min with subsequent centrifuging for 15 min at 2000 g. Supernatants were combined for subsequent immunochemical determination of apoA-I [27].

2.5. Isolation of Lipoproteins, Production of Apolipoprotein A-I

The study was carried out with Wistar rats weighing 180–200 g. Lipoproteins of blood serum were isolated by ultracentrifugation after chylomicrones removal from the blood serum [28]. Four main fractions of lipoproteins were obtained: VLDL ($0.94 < d < 1.006$ g/ml), LDL ($1.006 < d < 1.063$ g/ml), HDL_2 ($1.063 < d < 1.125$ g/ml), and HDL_3 ($1.125 < d < 1.21$ g/ml). Further the HDL_3 fraction was used. Delipidation of HDL was conducted with a cooled chloroform-methanol mixture (1:1), which was followed by multiple ether washing. An apo-HDL mixture was deposited over the column (1.6×100 cm) with 6B-CL Sepharose (Pharmacia, Sweden) and eluted with 0.01 M Tris-HCl buffer, pH 8.6, containing 6 M urea, 0.01% sodium azide, and 1 mM phenylmethylsulfonyl fluoride (PMSF). Elution profile was recorded from a UV detector 2151 LKB (Sweden). The purity of apoA-I was tested by electrophoresis in polyacrylamide gel (PAAG) with sodium dodecylsulphate (SDS) [24]. Apolipoprotein A-I formed a single band as a homogeneous 28 kDa protein. Protein bands were visualized with 0.1% Coomassie G-250 solution in the mixture of methanol and 10% acetic acid (1:1). Protein concentration in the samples was measured according to Lowry [22].

2.6. Isolation of Liver Cells, Analysis of DNA and Protein Synthesis in Hepatocytes

Liver cells were isolated after recirculation perfusion of the organ with a 0.03 % solution of collagenase-I (Boehringer Mannheim, Germany), as described earlier [29]. Hepatocytes were separated from nonparenchymal cells (NPC) by differential centrifugation with a centrifuge J2-21 (Beckman, USA). $(38 \pm 3) \cdot 10^6$ hepatocytes and $(40 \pm 3) \cdot 10^6$ NPC were isolated from 1 g of rat liver. Nonparenchymal cells were fractionated in a JE-6 elutriator rotor at 2500 rpm. Endotheliocytes and Kupffer cells were washed using the buffer elution rate of 22 and 42 ml/min, respectively. Cell counting was performed in a Goryaev chamber.

Cell viability was evaluated by Tripan Blue exclusion test. It was shown that more than 90% hepatocytes and 95% NPC to be viable. The obtained hepatocytes were resuspended in 5 ml Krebs-Ringer phosphate buffer to give 2-3 mg cell protein per 1 ml buffer. The cells were incubated over 24-hole Linbro plane-tables (Germany) with collagen-I support for 24 hours. Tetrahydrocortisol (THC) was added into incubation medium with concentration 10^{-6} M, apoA-I and its complex with THC – with concentration 70 mkg/ml. The complex was obtained via incubation of apoA-I and THC in 10 mM Tris-HCl buffer, pH 8.6, with the molar ratio 1:2, for 5 minutes at room temperature. The rate of DNA synthesis was determined by incorporation of ^{3}H-thymidine, while the rate of protein biosynthesis – by incorporation of ^{14}C-leucine. In both cases, concentration of tracer in the culture medium was 37 kBk/ml. To measure the DNA radioactivity the cells were transferred to a GF/C filter and washed out successively with 10% trichloracetic acid (TCA) and 95% ethanol. To measure the protein radioactivity the cells were transferred to a FN-16 filter pretreated with 0.1 M leucine solution in 10% TCA solution. Then the filters were washed out successively with TCA solution and ethanol-ether mixture. The samples radioactivity was measured with a fluid-scintillation counter Mark-III (USA). Radioactivity was calculated in impulses per minute per a hole.

2.7. Determination of Lipoprotein Binding Ability of the Cells

The obtained LDL (d = 1.019 – 1.063 g/ml) and HDL (d = 1.063 – 1.210 g/ml) were labeled with ^{125}I using a LodoGen preparation (Sigma, USA) [30]. Specific radioactivity of ^{125}I LP was 100 – 300 imp/ng of LP protein. More than 97% of radioactivity was precipitated by 10% trichloracetic acid. To estimate the LP binding ability, cells were incubated at 0°C in medium 199 containing 0.4% albumin and various concentrations of ^{125}I LP (3-80 µg/ml). Specific binding was calculated as the difference between amounts of ^{125}I LP bound to the cells in a 50-fold excess of unlabeled LP and in their absence; the obtained value was expressed as ng LP protein per 10^6 cells. The protein content in LP and isolated cells was determined by the Lowry [22]. Statistical processing of data was made using t-Student's test.

2.8. Choice of Interaction Sites between THC-ApoA-I Complex and DNA

The mechanism of activation of protein synthesis with participation of THC-apoA-I complex defines the processes of cell regeneration [15]. It means that this mechanism is associated with the concurrent expression of many genes. It follows that the DNA regulatory regions, sensitive to the action of the complex, must be widespread in the cell genome. The potential *cis*-element of the GCC-type meets these requirements. Computer search over the data base of mammalian nucleotide sequences (GenBank, EMBL DNA library) revealed the presence of a sequence of $CC(GCC)_n$ type at the Mer22 elements of DNA in primates [31]. The same sequence (only with a greater number of iterations) was found in the regulatory region of many mammalian and human genes. The 5′ flanking sequence of Homo sapiens multidrug resistence protein gene is an example [32]. In our study, a similar sequence was chosen for specificity analysis of interaction with tetrahydrocortisol-apoA-I complex. For comparison, a fragment of kDNA - regulatory region of cytochrome P-450 gene and oligonucleotide T_{19} were used. Primary structures of oligonucleotides were as follows:

1. 5′-CCGCCGCCGCCGCCGCC-3′
2. 5′-ATCTTTAACTGATGAACTTCT-3′
3. 5′-TTTTTTTTTTTTTTTTTTT-3′

Synthesis of all three oligonucleotides was conducted at the Federal Research Center of virology and biotechnology "Vector", Ministry of Health, Russian Federation. Cortisol (Serva, Germany) was used in the study, and its reduced form, tetrahydrocortisol, was kindly gifted by Academician Yu.A. Pankov (Russian Academy of Medical Sciences, Institute of experimental endocrinology, Moscow). Complexes of glucocorticoids with apoA-I were obtained by keeping their 2:1 molar ratio mixture in 0.05 M K-phosphate buffer, pH 7.4, for 5 min at room temperature. It`s ability to form the complexes was demonstrated previously [33]. The formation of the complex occurs very fast because the steroid hormones readily interact with the hydrophobic surface of the amphipatic regions of apolipoprotein A-I. Its K_{ass} is equal to $(0.4 \pm 0.1) \cdot 10^6$ M^{-1} and is significantly higher for HDL - $(2.0 \pm 0.2) \cdot 10^6$ M^{-1}, that is probably related with the influence of lipids on the protein conformation. The preparation of DNA-dependent RNA-polymerase (RNA-PM) of T7 phage was isolated from *E. coli* strain containing a cloned gene of RNA-polymerase from bacteriophage T7. Its purity was no less than 90% according to the data of electrophoresis under denaturating conditions.

2.9. Small-Angle X-Ray Scattering (SAXS)

SAXS is very sensitive and precise physical method for analyzing the structural changes in macromolecules and examining their interactions in the solution and the kinetics of these processes. The potentialities of this method in studying the structural changes in biological macromolecules still remain far being exhausted.

The SAXS method was used to estimate the effects of interaction of eukaryotic DNA and three synthetic single-chain oligonucleotides with the THC-apoA-I complex. Small-angle X-ray patterns were measured with a Siemens diffractometer (Germany). Wave length of X-ray radiation $\lambda = 0.154$ nm (CuK_α). Homogeneous preparations of apoA-I, RNA-PM, DNA and oligonucleotides with initial concentrations of 0.40, 1.52, 3.12, and 4.16 mg/ml, respectively, were used. To study the interaction effects of the native DNA with RNA-PM in the presence of apoA-I, mixtures of solutions of DNA, RNA-PM, apoA-I and complexes of apoA-I with glucocorticoids (cortisol and THC) of various concentrations were prepared preliminarily. Upon measuring the SAXS patterns, temperature of the initial preparations was 20°C, while that of DNA and RNA-PM mixtures was 37°C. To examine the interaction of oligonucleotides with apoA-I, mixtures of solutions of oligonucleotides with apoA-I and its complexes with glucocorticoids of various concentrations were prepared. Small-angle X-ray patterns were measured over the angle range $0.0245 \leq h \leq 3.423$ nm^{-1}, where $h = 4\pi\sin(\theta)/\lambda$, 2θ is the scattering angle. In the SAXS experimental data corrections were made for background scattering and collimation, the X-ray plots were smoothed.

3. Results

3.1. Mechanisms of Cell Proliferation after PLR and Their Relation with the Activity of Resident Macrophages

Reparative regeneration after liver resection is accompanied by a sharp enhancement of biosynthesis and functional activity of the remnant tissue. Liver is the organ which role in maintaining homeostasis in the organism can hardly be overstressed. Synthesis of lipids, detoxication of xenobiotics, metabolism of hormones, and many other processes are closely related with liver function. Pronounced deviations in homeostasis could be expected to occur after removing 2/3 of the organ; however, that is not the case. Actually, the remnant 1/3 takes up function of the whole organ. For example, the blood content of total lipids, phospholipids and triglycerides was shown to remain virtually constant in the dynamics of reparative liver regeneration [34]. Content of the total LDL and VLDL fraction increased progressively. This indicates the important role of LDL and VLDL in proliferative processes after hepatectomy (Table 1). Analysis of the lipoprotein spectrum of blood serum performed by electrophoresis in polyacrylamide gel revealed not only an increase in the amount of LDL and VLDL, but also a decrease in the concentration of HDL, mainly at the expense of HDL_3 fraction (Table 2). Thus, activation of proliferative processes in liver after its partial resection proceeded against the background of intense HDL_3 consumption. This mechanism is strongly contributed by glucocorticoids. As shown in our earlier work, injection of hydrocortisone to experimental animals increased the accumulation of VLDL in blood [35]. A certain dynamics of the blood content of glucocorticoids in rat after hepatectomy was found (Table 1). Thus, the blood concentration of 11-OCS sharply increased (560±32 μg/l) half an hour after the surgery. Tissue damage was perceived by the organism as acute stress. However, within 3 h the 11-OCS concentration reliably decreased, in a weak it approached the control level, and in 3 days became lower than control. So rapid decrease in the blood content of glucocorticoids at incomplete reparative process indicates that they are under close monitoring for stimulation of proliferative processes in liver.

Table 1. Effect of LPS on the blood serum content of glucocorticoids and total fraction of LDL and VLDL in intact and hepatectomized rats (M ± m)

Parameter	Control	Time after LPS injection or PLR, h			
		24	32-36	48	72
	1	2	3	4	5
Injection of LPS to intact animals					
11-OCS, μg/l	138.0±4.8	70.0±13.7	62.0±6.2	68.0±6.0	78.0±13.7
	(5)	(5)	(5)	(5)	(5)
Differences		$P_{1-2} < 0.05$	$P_{1-3} < 0.05$	$P_{1-4} < 0.05$	$P_{1-5} < 0.05$
LDL + VLDL, g/l	1.1±0.21	1.2±0.18	1.8±0.15	1.2±0.17	0.5±0.92
Differences			$P_{1-3} < 0.05$		
Hepatectomy					
11-OCS, mg/l	138.0±4.8	161.6±17.7	141.0±17.0	142.0±25.0	117.6±22.9
	(5)	(5)	(8)	(5)	(9)
LDL + VLDL, g/l	1.1±0.21	1.4±0.11	2.4±0.19	2.5±0.40	1.90±0.21
Differences			$P_{1-3} < 0.01$	$P_{1-4} < 0.01$	$P_{1-5} < 0.05$
Injection of LPS 24 h before PLR					
11-OCS, μg/l	138.0±4.8	83.2±9.5*	67.5±12.0*	68.8±12.0*	53.4±15.2*
		(5)	(9)	(5)	(7)
LDL + VLDL, g/l	1.1±0.21	2.3±0.11*	2.7±0.19	3.2±0.40	1.8±0.21

Note. An asterisk denotes reliable differences with respect to animals with PLR, which were not stimulated by LPS ($P < 0.05$).

Rapid activation of lysosomal apparatus of Kupffer macrophages in hepatectomized animals suggests that it is based on the active consumption (endocytosis) both of glucocorticoids and HDL_3 (the cooperative effect) with subsequent formation of heterophagolysosomes. This relationship was reported in our earlier work [34]. Stimulation of macrophages with LPS 24 h before the resection provided a more pronounced decrease in the blood content of 11-OCS and a more substantial increase in the total fraction of LDL and VLDL (Table 1). This circumstance may be related directly to a very rapid increase in the activity of lysosomal enzymes not only in macrophages, but also in hepatocytes, as well as to translocation of lysosomes to the cell nucleus and its preparation to mitosis. The dependence of these processes on LPS stimulation of Kupffer macrophages or their blocking with colloidal iron is demonstrated below.

Table 2. Effect of PLR and LPS stimulation of macrophages on lipoproteins spectrum of rat blood serum %

Conditions of experiment	HDL_2	HDL_3	LDL	VLDL
Intact animals (17)	28.8±1.48	51.3±1.95	16.0±1.25	4.0±0.62
After PLR:				
In 12 h (n=5)	48.2±2.8	9.4±9.80	20.9±7.50	21.4±5.50
In 32 h (n=5)	29.9±4.60	11.0±4.20	31.1±6.30	27.2±2.80
After LPS injection:				
In 24 h (n=16)	35.9±1.68*	42.1±2.04*	16.7±1.20	5.3±0.91
In 48 h (n=5)	47.7±3.00*	35.2±3.80*	6.3±1.30	10.7±1.30

* - difference ($P < 0.05$) from intact animals; column 1 (n) – number of animals.

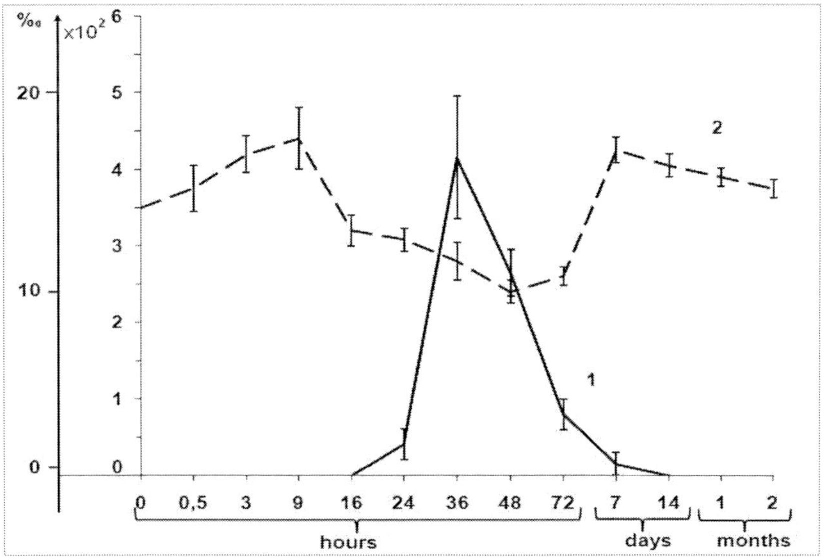

Figure 1. The number of hepatocyte mitoses (1) and relative content of Kupffer cells (2) after PLR [34]. *Absciss*: time after operation. *Ordinate*: left scale — **hepatocyte mitoses, ‰; right scale** — the number of Kupffer cells per 1000 hepatocytes × 10^2.

The single dividing hepatocytes could be seen as early as 24 h after PLR. At 36 hours maximal mitotic activity was revealed (2.24 ± 0.02%). 48 and 72 h after an operation hepatocyte mitotic rate decreased from 1.2 ± 0.8% to 0.27 ± 0.01% (Fig. 1).

In control liver slice was 371 ± 4.2 Kupffer cells per 1000 hepatocytes. 2.5 h after PLR their amount increased up to 413 ± 6.3 per 1000 hepatocytes ($P < 0.01$) and 9 h after the operation their mean relative value was 21.7% greater than in controls ($P < 0.01$). Later, during premitotic and mitotic reriods, i.e. at 24 and 36 h, the relative number of Kupffer cells fell down to 318 ± 8.1 and 258.0 ± 4.5. At 48 h this value tended to increase again, but at 72 h it remained significantly lower than in controls ($P < 0.01$) (Fig. 1).

It was shown that PLR led to changes of lysosomal enzyme activities in Kupffer cell fraction (Fig. 2). The total lysosomal enzyme activities in Kupffer sells increased 1.5 - 2.5 fold within the first hours of postoperative period. Thus 2.5 h after PLR the asid DNA-ase activity was 65% greater than in control liver ($P < 0.05$). Acid RNA-ase was 130 - 140% and cathepsin D activity 30% greater than those of Kupffer cells from sham-operated controls. The high total lysosomal hydrolase activities in Kupffer cells were maintained through the first 24 h after an operation. Towards 36 h the DNA-ase and cathepsin D activities decreased, but the total acid RNA-ase activity remained at high level comparing controls at every point after PLR.

2.5 h after the operation the 1.5 - 3 fold increase of free lysosomal hydrolase activities in liver macrophages could be seen. At 9 h free acid DNA-ase and acid RNA-ase activities decreased, while the cathepsin D activity kept almoust 2-fold greater than in controls ($P < 0.01$). At 24 h the free activity of any enzyme reversed to control level. At 36 h maximum mitotic activity only traces of asid DNA-ase activity could be detected. At 72 h the secondary slight increase of free acid RNA-ase and cathepsin D activities was found while only trace amounts of acid DNA-ase activity could be detected.

The phase fluctuations of total lysosomal activities in hepatocytes corresponded well with their outchanges in whole liver extracts. Worth to be mentioned the moderate increase of total DNA-ase and RNA-ase activities 9 h after PLR. Later, the increase gave up to decrease of acid DNA-ase and other enzymes activities. It was most obvious 24 h after PLR, i.e. at the moment of greatest DNA synthesis in hepatocytes, and 36 h after operation when maximal hepatocyte mitotic activity was observed. The total cathepsin D activity was lower than in controls ($P < 0.05$). Later the lysosomal enzyme activities rised again. At 72 h the total DNA-ase activity was 28% and that of RNA-ase – 23% greater than in sham-operated rats.

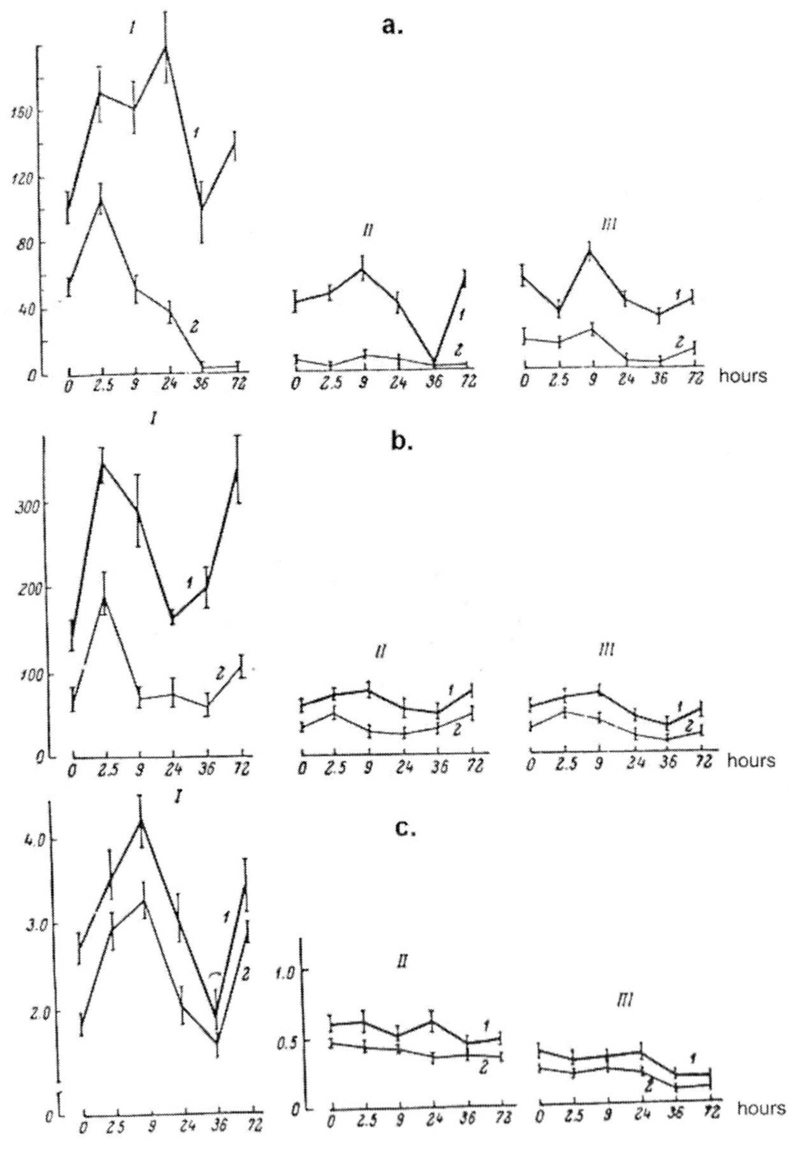

Figure 2. Total (1) and free (2) lysosomal enzyme activities during liver regeneration after partial liver removal. a - acid DNA–ase, b - acid RNA-ase, c - cathepsin D. I - Kupffer cells, II - hepatocytes, III - whole liver homogenate. *Absciss:* time after operation in hours. *Ordinate* : a, b - released AMP, micromole per mg protein/hour, c - **values of ΔE per 30 min, %**;. *Vertical bars*: standart error deviations.

The free acid RNA-ase activity increased while that of acid DNA-ase – decreased 2.5 h after PLR. At 9 h the reverse correlations between both enzymes could be seen. Later only trace values of free acid DNA-ase activity were found while other activities were around control figures (Fig. 2).

The importance of Kupffer cells in liver regeneration is supported in following experiments. Liver regeneration was studied under Kupffer cell blockade. The blockade or functional elimination of liver macrophages was performed by means of intravenous injection of 1 ml of 5% suspension of colloidal iron 2 h before, 3 or 18 h after PLR, i.e. at two different points of hepatocytes proliferation – at the beginning and in the heat of DNA synthesis. In control series starch-stabilized colloidal carbon was replaced with starch solution without inert colloid. When Kuppfer cells were eliminated immediately before an operation or 3 h after PLR the hepatocyte proliferation was delayed. In these livers mitosis appeared as late as 32 h after PLR and maximum mitotic rate could be found not earlier than 48 h after liver mass removal. At the same time the well-defined mitotic "tail" resisted up to 72 h while in controls the mitotic activity at this time-point was considerably less. When colloidal iron was injected 18 h after PLR the dynamics of mitoses was alike that in control series though peak-amplitude at 32 h was less than in controls (Fig. 3).

So, when Kupffer cells were overloaded with inert colloid particles the mitotic patterns were changed. The most remarkable finding was the delay and decrease in amplitude of hepatocyte mitotic peak when blockade was performed 3 h after PLR, but not 18 h after it (Fig. 3).

Perhaps the overloading of liver macrophages with foreign deposits at the early stages of regeneration most effectively modifies interrelations between Kupffer cells and hepatocytes as a part of stromal-parenchymatous morphogenic ties. The modification may be attributed to many reasons though its exact nature remains unknown. We are inclined to suppose that one of the most important points lays within changes of macrophage secretory functions due to their overloading. It is very probable that overloaded Kupffer cells have lost temporarily or constantly the ability to secret lysosomal hydrolases, the triggers of intrahepatic growth.

On the contrary, injection of LPS drastically enhanced the regenerative activity of hepatocytes. This showed up as an earlier initiation of DNA synthesis and appearance of hepatocyte mitoses and also as a more synchronous start of mitotic division of hepatocytes (Table 3). Thus, an increased mitotic activity in non-stimulated animals was recorded 24 h after the surgery; then the activity rose sharply with a peak at 30-36 h. In rats stimulated with LPS, the peak of mitotic activity was higher as compared to that in the first group of animals, and occurred earlier, within 24 h after PLR.

Absciss: time after partial liver removal (PLR) in hours. *Ordinate*: mitoses per 1000 hepatocytes. a, b, c: colloidal iron was injected 2 h before, 3 and 18 h after PLR. 1: mitoses under overloading, 2: mitoses in control rats. *Vertical bars*: standard error deviations.

As was noted above, Kupffer macrophages can be involved in the regulation of liver regeneration process by different ways. In our case, most essential is that mononuclear phagocytes secrete a set of biologically active substances, in particular lysosomal enzymes, into the intercellular medium. The enzymes, coming to the medium from activated macrophages, can exert a stimulating action on proliferation of hepatocytes. This can explain why stimulation of macrophages by bacterial polysaccharides in our experiments substantially accelerated the liver regeneration.

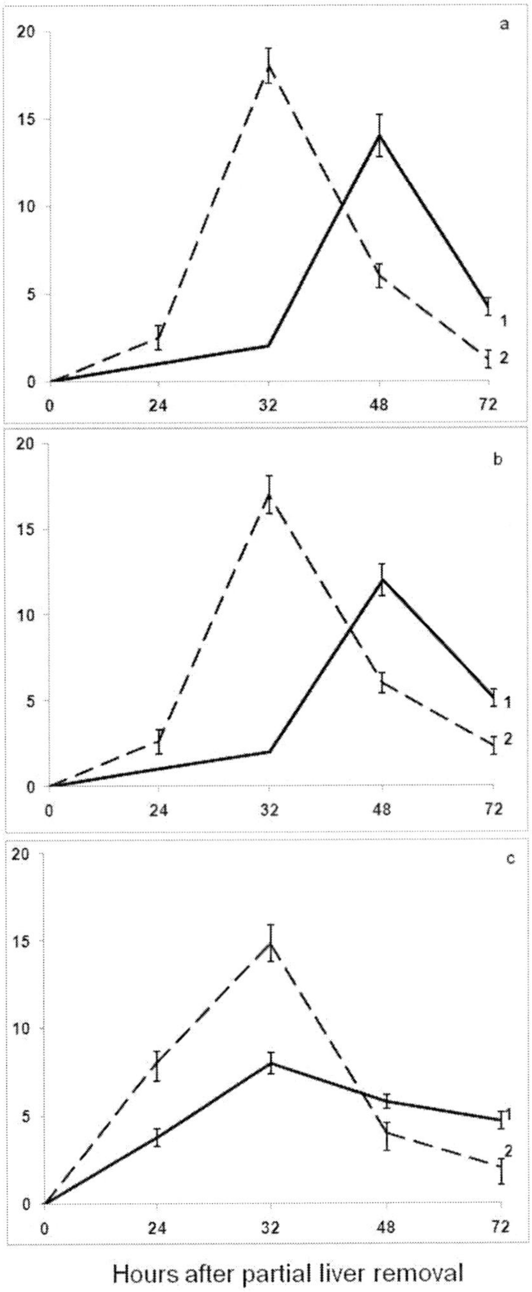

Figure 3. Hepatocyte mitotic activity under Kupffer cell blockade.

Earlier [36], it was shown that Kupffer cells stimulated in vitro by bacterial polysaccharide start to synthesize intensely and secrete into the incubation medium lysozyme, plasminogen activator, procoagulants, acid phosphatase, and β- glucuronidase. The activated macrophages can secrete also glucosidases into the medium. Glucosidases are capable of splitting the structural glycoproteins in the plasmatic membrane of the target cells, in particular fibronectin, which provides coupling of the cells and prevents their proliferation. Besides, lysosomal enzymes (proteinases) from extracellular medium can be involved in a cascade mechanism starting with the activation of serine proteinase bound to the plasmatic membrane of the target cell. This induces a series of cell events resulting in the transformation of a resting cell into proliferating one. We observed translocation of lysosomes to the perinuclear region of hepatocytes and their contact with the nuclear membrane within 9 hours after PLR. 24 h after PLR, contours of the nuclei were blurred (Fig. 4). A similar mechanism was initiated in the surviving rat liver sections upon their incubation with HDL and cortisol (Fig. 5). This was accompanied by activation of chromatin and enhancement of AO binding to DNA (Table 4). Blocking of intracellular transfer of lysosomes by vinblastin or colchicine diminished the affinity of nuclear chromatin for AO to the control values. Similar results were obtained for the inhibition of proteolytic activity by gordox, pepstatin, iodoacetamide, and soybean inhibitor of trypsin. These facts testify that activation of lysosomes and their interaction with the nucleus in the early prereplicative period are closely related to initiation of cell division after PLR.

Table 3. Dynamics of mitotic activity of hepatocytes after stimulation of liver macrophage system with LPS (M ± m, n = 6), %

Time after PLR, h	Non-stimulated rats (control)	Stimulated rats (experiment)	P
20	rare mitosises	0.94 ± 0.062	< 0.01
24	0.31 ± 0.028	2.62 ± 0.097	< 0.01
30	2.07 ± 0.07	1.32 ± 0.071	< 0.01
36	1.57 ±.100	0.67 ± 0.052	< 0.01
48	0.68 ± 0.101	0.47 ± 0.033	> 0.05
72	0.18 ± 0.017	0.09 ± 0.038	> 0.05

Table 4. Molar concentration of AO binding sites (n_{sp}) in a suspension of nuclei isolated from the surviving rat liver sections incubated with hydrocortisone, HDL and lysosomal inhibitors (µmol/g protein, M ± m)

Control (no additives) + HDL	Hydro-cortisone + HDL	Hydrocortisone + HDL + vinblastin	Hydro-cortisone + HDL + colchicine	Hydro-cortisone + HDL + pepstatin	Hydro-cortisone + HDL + iodoacetamide	Hydro-cortisone + HDL + soybean inhibitor of trypsin
7.02 ± 0.54 (35)	13.76 ± 1.68** (25)	7.15 ± 1.14 (14)	7.59 ±1.48 (5)	8.26 ± 0.84 (10)	6.10 ± 1.03 (10)	6.93 ± 1.04 (9)

Note: ** P < 0.001 with respect to control.

Thus, using hepatectomized rats it was shown that immediately after partial liver removal the Kupffer macrophages were accumulated in liver remnant. At the maximal mitotic activity (36 hours following PLR) the relative amount of Kupffer cells keeps low, but 72 hours later turns out to be higher again. The periodic changes of the Kupffer cell amount in hepa tectomized rats are accompanied by remarkable increase (1.5 - 3 fold) of free and total lysosomal enzyme activity (acid DNA-ase, acid RNA-ase, cathepsin D). The activation of the

Kupffer macrophage lysosomes goes ahead of labilization of hepatocyte lysosomal membranes.

The blockade of mononuclear phagocyte system by means of carbonate iron overloading in the early prereplicative period leads to an as long as 10 - 12 hours retardation of hepatocyte proliferation. The role of Kupffer macrophages in reparative liver regeneration is very important.

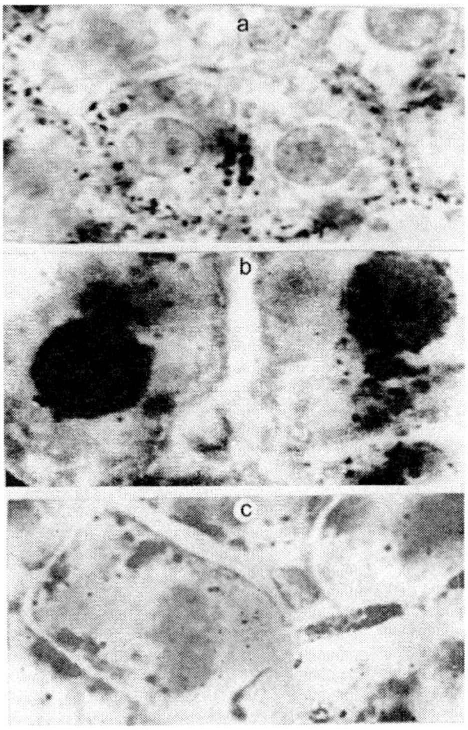

Figure 4. Changes in the activity of acid phosphatase in hepatocytes in different periods of reparative liver regeneration. a — control; b — 9 h after hepatectomy; c — 24 h after the surgery; Homory's stain, x 900.

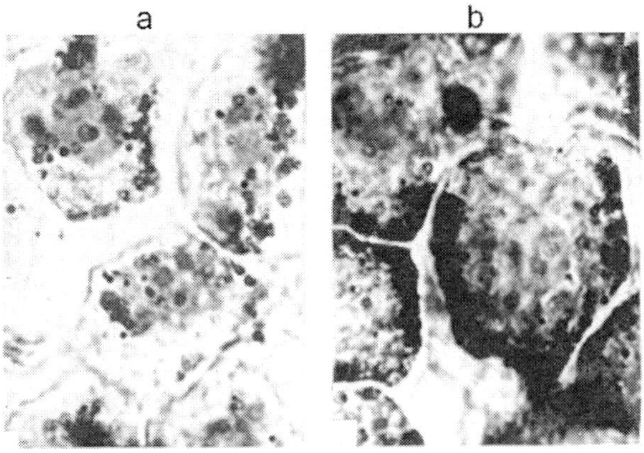

Figure 5. Activity of acid phosphatase in surviving rat liver sections upon their incubation with: a – hydrocortisone and HDL; b – hydrocortisone + HDL + vinblastin; Homory's stain, x 1000.

3.2. The Effect of Resident Macrophages on Protein and Apolipoprotein Biosynthesis in a Regenerating Liver

Cell regeneration is closely related to the enhancement of protein biosynthesis in a resected organ. We have demonstrated that this process depends to a great extent on the activity of resident macrophages.

Thus, 48 hours after the stimulation of resident macrophages by LPS, a significant enhancement of the protein synthesis rate occurred in both the homogenates and supernatants (Table 5).

Table 5. Influence of residential macrophages activation in the rate of ^{14}C-leucine incorporation into proteins in the livers of intact and hepatectomized rats, counts/min/mg protein (M ± m)

Group number	Experimental conditions	Homogenate	Supernatant
1	Control	4428 ± 285	4673 ± 385
2	LPS, 48 h before sacrifice	5716 ± 574	6020 ± 647
3	Sham-operation, 24 h before sacrifice	5111 ± 188	6377 ± 727
4	LPS + sham-operation	5235 ± 431	5679 ± 410
5	Partial liver removal (PLR), 24 h before sacrifice	7320 ± 756	6859 ± 568
6	LPS + PLR	9554 ± 586	8658 ± 547
	Differences between groups		
	Groups:	P <	P <
	1-2	0.05	0.05
	1-3	0.05	0.05
	1-4	0.05	0.05
	1-5	0.01	0.01
	1-6	0.01	0.01
	2-6	0.01	0.01
	3-5	0.05	-
	4-6	0.01	0.01
	5-6	0.05	0.05

The sham operation also increased incorporation of ^{14}C-leucine into total proteins of the liver homogenate and supernatant. In this case, the mechanism of protein synthesis enhancement is probably the same as in the LPS experiments: stimulation of the macrophages by autoantigens formed in the organism in response to tissue damage during the operation. This may be a reason why the sham-operated animals that were pretreated with LPS did not show a further increase in the rate of protein synthesis both in the homogenate and supernatant. One day after removal of 2/3 of the liver, there was a considerable increase in the protein synthesis rate in the remaining tissue: in the homogenate by 65%, and in the supernatant by 45%. Activation of the regenerative processes was preceded by an increase in the rate of protein synthesis.

Treatment of animals with LPS 24 hours before PLR led to a sharp increase in the rate of protein synthesis in the remaining tissue 24 hours after the operation: in the homogenate by 115% and in the supernatant by 85% (Table 5). This fact can probably explain why the maximum of mitotic activity shifted to 24 hours after the operation (see Table 3).

Thus, in comparison with the control (taken as 100%), the rate of protein synthesis increased under the influence of LPS alone by 129%; of PLR alone, by 165%; and due to combined action of LPS and PLR, by 215%. For the supernatants, an increase was equal to 128%, 146% and 185%, respectively. The data presented indicate that resident macrophages play an important role in the regulation of protein biosynthesis in the normal liver (intracellular regeneration).

We also examined incorporation of ^{14}C-leucine into the blood serum proteins after removal of lipoproteins. The corresponding radioactivities of the blood serum proteins were found: 1) control, 12846 ± 256.2; 2) after treatment of the animals with LPS, 15640 ± 2409; 3) after the sham operation, 14957 ± 1363; 4) after the sham operation of the animals pretreated with LPS, 15348 ± 589; 5) after partial hepatectomy (PLR), 15398 ± 1320; and 6) after hepatectomy of the animals pretreated with LPS, 15264 ± 1400 counts/min/mg of protein. In cases 4, 5, 6, changes were significant with respect to the control.

Thus, the in vivo stimulation of resident macrophages leads to an abrupt enhancement of protein biosynthesis in intact animals and in animals with PLR, and in this way promotes the proliferative processes in the liver. It should be emphasized that the stimulation increases the synthesis not only of proteins that are necessary for the restoration of integrity of the liver, but also the synthesis of proteins of the body's internal medium, i.e., the proteins which are "exported" from the liver to maintain the oncotic pressure of blood.

Lipoproteins (LDL and VLDL) are known to serve as a source of building material (cholesterol and phospholipids) in the dividing cells [18]. Macrophages also play a key role in lipoprotein metabolism [34].

We have found that the in vivo stimulation of the macrophages by LPS increased the incorporation of ^{14}C-leucine into the proteins of VLDL, LDL, HDL_2, and decreased its incorporation into the proteins of HDL_3. The sham operation caused similar effects, although changes in the protein synthesis in HDL_2 and HDL_3 were less pronounced (Table 6).

The sham operation performed after LPS treatment of the animals led to a further increase in the rates of protein biosynthesis in VLDL and LDL, but had no effect on the protein synthesis in HDL_2 and significantly decreased it in HDL_3. Partial hepatectomy in comparison with the control decreased the rate of ^{14}C-leucine incorporation into proteins of VLDL and HDL_3 and did not influence the protein synthesis in LDL and HDL_2. The partial hepatectomy performed 24 h after LPS treatment of the animals enhanced the protein synthesis in VLDL and LDL, but had no effect on the proteins of HDL_2 and HDL_3.

Our earlier studies revealed that cooperative capture of HDL_3 and steroid hormones (glucocorticoids) is connected with macrophages and proceeds via the receptor-mediated endocytosis [15, 29]. This conclusion was confirmed also by the present study on LPS stimulation of macrophages. A similar mechanism is initiated at PLR. Thus, preliminary stimulation of macrophages with LPS considerably improves the reparative potential of liver. This is strongly contributed by an increased secretion of LDL and VLDL by hepatocytes, which is related with acceleration of protein (apolipoprotein) biosynthesis in them. However, a decrease in the rate of protein biosynthesis in lipoproteins was observed in our work only after partial resection of liver. Such inhibition was more pronounced in VLDL. In LDL, where apoB-100 is the main protein, no inhibition was observed. This suggests that synthesis of the indicated protein in liver is controlled by a cooperative mechanism related with the action of HDL_3 and steroid hormones.

Table 6. Influence of the residential macrophages on the rate of ^{14}C-leucine incorporation into proteins of the blood lipoproteins, counts/min/mg protein (M ± m)

Group number	Experimental conditions	VLDL	LDL	HDL_2	HDL_3
1	Control	15101 ± 1438	22941 ± 191	11508 ± 2121	14652 ± 764
2	LPS	18775 ± 2547	33856 ± 1748	17191 ± 162	6428 ± 2189
3	Sham-operation	18755 ± 2209	30916 ± 2737	13974 ± 484	10551 ± 784
4	LPS + Sham-operation	22687 ± 191	39662 ± 3119	10003 ± 3146	6107 ± 1040
5	Partial liver removal (PLR)	8059 ± 540	23147 ± 461	10935 ± 2693	5657 ± 1238
6	LPS + PLR	12377 ± 1211	45384 ± 1879	7927 ± 2162	4770 ± 274
	Differences between groups				
	Groups:	P <	P <	P <	P <
	1-2	0.05	0.05	0.05	0.05
	1-3	0.05	0.05	-	0.05
	1-4	0.05	0.05	-	0.05
	1-5	0.01	0.05	-	0.05
	1-6	-	0.05	0.05	0.05
	2-4	-	0.05	0.05	-
	2-6	0.05	0.05	0.01	-
	3-4	0.05	0.05	-	0.05
	3-5	0.01	0.05	-	0.05
	4-6	0.01	0.05	-	0.05
	5-6	0.05	0.05	-	-

LPS stimulation of macrophages and partial liver resection produced different changes in the rate of protein synthesis in HDL_2 and HDL_3. In HDL_2 the rate either increased or showed no changes. In HDL_3 it was strongly inhibited in all cases. In both HDL fractions, the main proteins are represented by apoA-I and apoA-II. Two organs are known to be responsible for the synthesis of these proteins: liver and small intestines [37]. Our special studies revealed that initiation of the cooperative mechanism of HDL_3 and steroid hormones action, which is related with the enhancement of protein biosynthesis in liver, leads to concurrent inhibition of protein synthesis in other organs, for example, in the small intestines [38]. A possible explanation of the observed differences is that synthesis of apoA-I and apoA-II in HDL_2 is related mainly to liver, whereas that in HDL_3 — to the small intestines.

Binding and the subsequent uptake of lipoproteins by macrophages (endothelial cells and hepatocytes) through receptor-mediated endocytosis was also investigated in this work. Thus, the number of receptors on the surface of macrophages activated by LPS should decrease and, hence, binding of labeled HDL should also decrease. We showed that 24 h after administration of LPS the binding of ^{125}I HDL by Kupffer's cells decreased 4.5-fold. This was recovered after 72 h, but the initial level was not attained. No significant changes in the binding of ^{125}I HDL by endothelial cells was observed. Quite different dynamics were observed with hepatocytes. The increase in binding of ^{125}I HDL was 1.2-fold after 24 h and 2.2-fold after 72 h (Fig. 6).

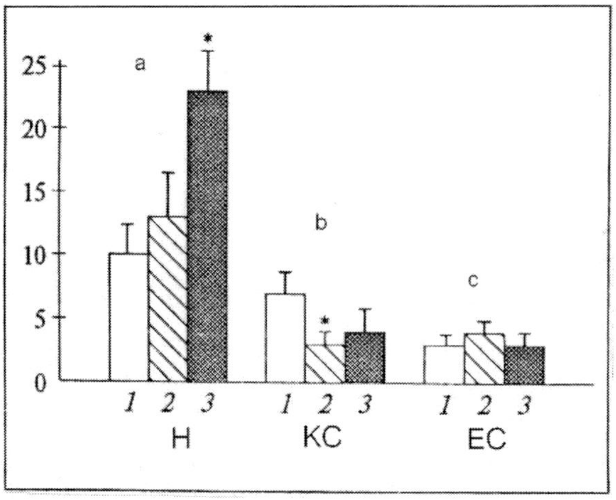

Figure 6. Effect of LPS-induced stimulation of macrophages on the binding of ^{125}I HDL to hepatocytes (a), Kupffer's cells (b), and endothelial cells (c): 1) control; 2) 24-h stimulation; 3) 72-h stimulation. H – hepatocytes, KC - Kupffer's cells, EC - endothelial cells. ** - $p < 0.01$.

The results obtained give grounds to state that LPS-activated macrophages can capture HDL via the receptor-mediated endocytosis. Receptor internalization diminishes binding of ^{125}I HDL within 24 h after the stimulation. Restoration of HDL binding proceeds slowly and remains incomplete in 72 h. However, this induces a mechanism that enhances the growth of receptors on hepatocytes, the number of receptors doubling by 72 h. If macrophages capture HDL together with cortisol, this leads to the formation and subsequent secretion of biologically active complex THC-apoA-I. The latter is captured by hepatocytes to enhance gene expression and protein synthesis rate in them. The indicated increase in the number of receptors in hepatocytes within 72 h can also be attributed to this mechanism.

3.3. The Effect of Cortisol (THC)-ApoA-I Complex on In Vitro Biosynthesis of Protein and DNA in the Liver Cells

This work demonstrated that THC-apoA-I complex exhibited biological activity only in parenchymal cells, whereas cortisol-apoA-I complex had no effect on hepatocytes and hepatic sinusoidal cells.

This is indicated by results of incubation of hepatocytes, Kupffer cells, and endotheliocytes with steroid hormones, apoA-I and their complexes (Table 7). As shown, cortisol and tetrahydrocortisol did not enhance the protein biosynthesis rate in any type of cells, whereas apoA-I was proved to increase significantly the rate of ^{14}C-leucine incorporation only in Kupffer cells. Also, the complex cortisol+apoA-I insignificantly inhibited the protein biosynthesis in hepatocytes. On the contrary, the complex THC+apoA-I enhanced largely the synthesis of proteins in the cells. The results obtained indicate that reduced forms of steroid hormones (tetrahydrocortisol) are biologically active and they regulate gene expression in liver parenchymal cells. A similar mechanism operates also in a regenerating liver and leads to DNA reduplication.

Table 7. Action of the apoA-I, cortisol, and tetrahydrocortisol (THC) on the rate of protein biosynthesis in cultures of hepatocytes, macrophages, and hepatic endothelial cells (M ± m)

Experimental conditions	Rate of ^{14}C-leucine incorporation into a protein (counts/min per 1 well)		
	Hepatocytes	Macrophages	Endothelial cells
Control	3492 ± 71	1420 ± 102	1580 ± 193
Cortisol	3190 ± 62	1381 ± 135	1474 ± 192
THC	3630 ± 122^{b}	1540 ± 312	1220 ± 190
ApoA-I	3840 ± 93^{a,b}	2790 ± 420^{a}	1636 ± 175
Cortisol + apoA-I	3083 ± 60^{a}	1832 ± 193	1550 ± 84
THC + apoA-I	4860 ± 503^{a}	1890 ± 390	1350 ± 302

Each experiment was repeated 5 -10 times. a – P <0.05 compared with control; b – P <0.05 compared with the group THC+apoA-I.

Table 8. Changes in DNA biosynthesis rate in the organs and tissues of mice after partial liver resection at in vivo stimulation of mononuclear phagocyte system with LPS (M ± m; n = 6)

Organs and tissues	Incorporation of ^{3}H-thymidine into DNA, imp/min per 1 μg DNA			
	Control	PLR	LPS	PLR+LPS
Liver	75±7	146±12	94±9*	185±32*∇◊
Bone marrow	1018±135	606±89*	766±194	693±62
Small intestines	821 ±97	373±129*	658±19	651±18

* — a reliable difference from the control (P < 0.05); # — between PLR and LPS groups (P < 0.05); ∇ — between LPS and PLR + LPS groups (P < 0.05); ◊ — between PLR and PLR + LPS groups (P < 0.05).

The rate of DNA synthesis in a regenerating liver was shown to increase twofold 24 h after hepatectomy. Stimulation of Kupffer cells by LPS leads to its further increase (Table 8). This shifts the mitotic activity of hepatocytes to an earlier period (Table 3). An opposite pattern was observed in the small intestines and red bone marrow: DNA synthesis was suppressed. The suppression was caused by the preferential capture of HDL_3 and glucocorticoids by macrophages of the regenerating liver. It is supposed that in other tissues a similar mechanism was concurrently inhibited. Cortisol plays a key role in the enhancement of DNA synthesis. This is demonstrated by the studies where the hormone is added to the macrophage-hepatocyte co-culture in a complex with apoA-I or HDL_3 (Table 9). Here, the role of macrophage consists in fast reduction of Δ^4,3-ketogroup of the hormone A ring with the formation of THC. The THC complex with apoA-I is active form of the hormone, which is capable of initiating DNA synthesis. The results obtained allow a conclusion that a similar mechanism operates in the dividing liver cells after PLR.

Thus, it was shown for the first time that the reduced form of cortisol, tetrahydrocortisol, is the biologically active form of hormone. It contributes to the stimulation of both the protein and DNA biosynthesis in liver cells (hepatocytes). However, this effect appears only when the hormone forms a complex with apolipoprotein A-I. Here apoA-I acts as a targeted carrier of hormone to the cells nuclei for its further interaction with certain sites of deproteinized DNA regions. We verified this hypothesis using the small-angle X-ray scattering technique.

Table 9. Effect of THC-apoA-I complex on the rate of DNA and protein biosynthesis in hepatocytes

Incubation conditions	Incorporation if ^{3}H-thymidine into DNA, imp/min/per hole		Incorporation of ^{14}C-leucine into protein (counts/min per hole)	
	Without apoA-I	With apoA-I	Without apoA-I	With apoA-I
Control	4459 ± 157	3320 ± 511	760 ± 34.7	386 ± 21.1
Tetrahydrocortisol	3393 ± 333^{a}	4928 ± 115^{a+}	692 ± 34.7	1098 ± 107.4^{a+}

^{a} – *Reliable distinctions compared to the corresponding control.*
$^{+}$ - ***Compared to the parameters*** *"without apoA-I". P <0.05.*

3.4. Molecular Mechanisms of DNA Reduplication during Cell Division

Previously, the SAXS method was successfully used in our study on interaction of specific tRNA with tRNA-synthetases [39], of oligonucleotides with methyltransferases [40], in evaluating the structural changes in HDL [41]. SAXS was proven useful in studying the mechanisms of molecular interaction, in particular, allowing one to analyze stoichiometry and equilibrium constants of macromolecular complexes, structural and weight properties of macromolecules. Fig. 7a shows the SAXS plots obtained for RNA-PM preparations, DNA (Fig. 7b), and apoA-I (Fig. 7c), and their mixtures with apoA-I and glucocorticoids (Fig. 8a). Radius of gyration (Rg) value for RNA-PM of T7 phage (Rg = 6.83 ± 0.15 nm) obtained from the SAXS data is close to the value (Rg = 6.6 ± 0.3 nm) reported for β′-subunit of RNA-PM from *E. coli* by other authors [42]. DNA and apoA-I structures were described in our work previously [43]. Free DNA in a solution is known to take the shape of Gaussian ball [44] with cavities filled by a solvent. Thus, the value of radius of gyration Rg = 39.2 ± 0.5 nm, obtained by SAXS for the native DNA isolated from rat liver, reflects a full volume filled with a knot of DNA double chain with inflections, and molecular mass estimated at $26 \cdot 10^{6}$ kDa agrees well with the literature data [45]. The DNA structure used in this work is presented in Table 10.

Table 10. Structural and mass parameters of native DNA from rat liver estimated using SAXS

R_g(nm)	R (nm)	$V \cdot 10^{-3}$ (nm^{3})	$M_s \cdot 10^{-6}$ (Da)^{2}	$M_s \cdot 10^{-6}$ (Da)^{2}	$M_s \cdot 10^{-6}$ (Da)
39.0 ± 0.5	50.3	533	482	26.0 ± 2.0	27.0 ± 5.0

V, R are the volume and radius of the sphere, respectively. $^{a}M_p = V\rho_0/1.66$ *(Da)*, where $\rho_0 = 1.5$ g/cm^{3}.

To assess the effects of RNA-PM and apoA-I interaction with DNA by SAXS, equilibrium mixtures of RNA-PM and DNA with apoA-I and its complexes with tetrahydrocortisol were used. Fig. 8 and Tables 11 and 12 present the SAXS plots and list the values of structural characteristics of scattering particles obtained from DNA preparation and DNA mixtures with RNA-PM and apoA-I in the presence and in the absence of THC.

Table 11. Average values of radius of gyration (R_g) and intensities of X-ray scattering to the zero angle ($I(0)$) obtained from the SAXS data, at molar concentrations of RNA-PM (C_p) and DNA (C_s) in the presence (+) and in the absence (-) of THC and apoA-I in the mixtures

THC	ApoA-I	C_p (mkM)	C_s (mkM)	R_g (nm)	$I(0)$ (imp/s)
-	-	-	0.043	39.1 ± 0.5	1450 ± 11
-	-	0.140	0.043	38.8 ± 0.7	1485 ± 15
-	3.55	0.140	0.043	39.3 ± 0.6	1490 ± 12
+	3.55	-	0.043	39.2 ± 0.4	1605 ± 10

Table 12. Average values of radius of gyration (R_g), intensities of X-ray scattering to the zero angle ($I(0)$), and the number of RNA-PM molecules (n) in P*n*S complexes obtained from the SAXS data, at molar concentrations of apoA-I, RNA-PM (C_p) and DNA (C_s) in the mixtures

Mixture	ApoA-I (mkM)	C_p (mkM)	C_s (mkM)	R_g (nm)	$I(0)$ (imp/s)	n	C_p/C_s
1	3.55	0.140	0.043	39.0 ± 0.6	1764 ± 5	2	3
2	3.55	0.238	0.043	38.9 ± 0.7	1881 ± 7	4	5
3	3.55	0.380	0.043	39.2 ± 0.5	1960 ± 8	5	9
4	3.55	0.568	0.043	39.7 ± 0.8	1988 ± 8	6	13

Measurements were made in the presence of THC in the mixtures. For the complex (DNA + apoA-I) at C_s = 0.043 mkM, I(0) = 1605 ± 9 imp/s

Values of Rg and $I(0)$ for various mixtures of apoA-I with DNA and RNA-PM were calculated from experimental data. One can see from Fig. 10 and Tables 11 and 12 that a marked interaction of DNA with apoA-I and RNA-PM was observed only in the THC presence. In the absence of THC small interaction of DNA with apoA-I and RNA-PM was observed. The size of P*n*S complexes (here P stands for RNA-PM; S denotes DNA aggregates with THC–apoA-I; n is the number of P molecules in the complex) within the accuracy of measurements corresponded to the size of DNA molecules in a free state (Rg = 39.2 ± 0.6 nm), while reliably changed only the values of $I(0)$ related to concentration and molecular mass of P*n*S complexes [39, 40]:

$$I(0) \sim \mathrm{N} \cdot \mathrm{M}^2, \qquad (1)$$

where N, M are, respectively the number and the mass of P*n*S complexes involved into scattering.

It is known that the integrity of secondary DNA structure can be judged from the occurrence of diffraction maximum in the angle range of h ~ 0.266 nm^{-1} [45] at the SAXS plot corresponding to the diameter of DNA double chain (~ 2.2 nm). One can see in Fig. 8 that at $h \approx 0.27 \pm 0.02$ nm^{-1} the diffraction maximum is clearly observed at SAXS plots from preparations of the native DNA and DNA mixtures with apoA-I without hormones, while with similar mixtures in the presence of THC the peak value decreases reliably. This indicates the rupture of secondary DNA structure in the process of DNA interaction with THC-apoA-I complex.

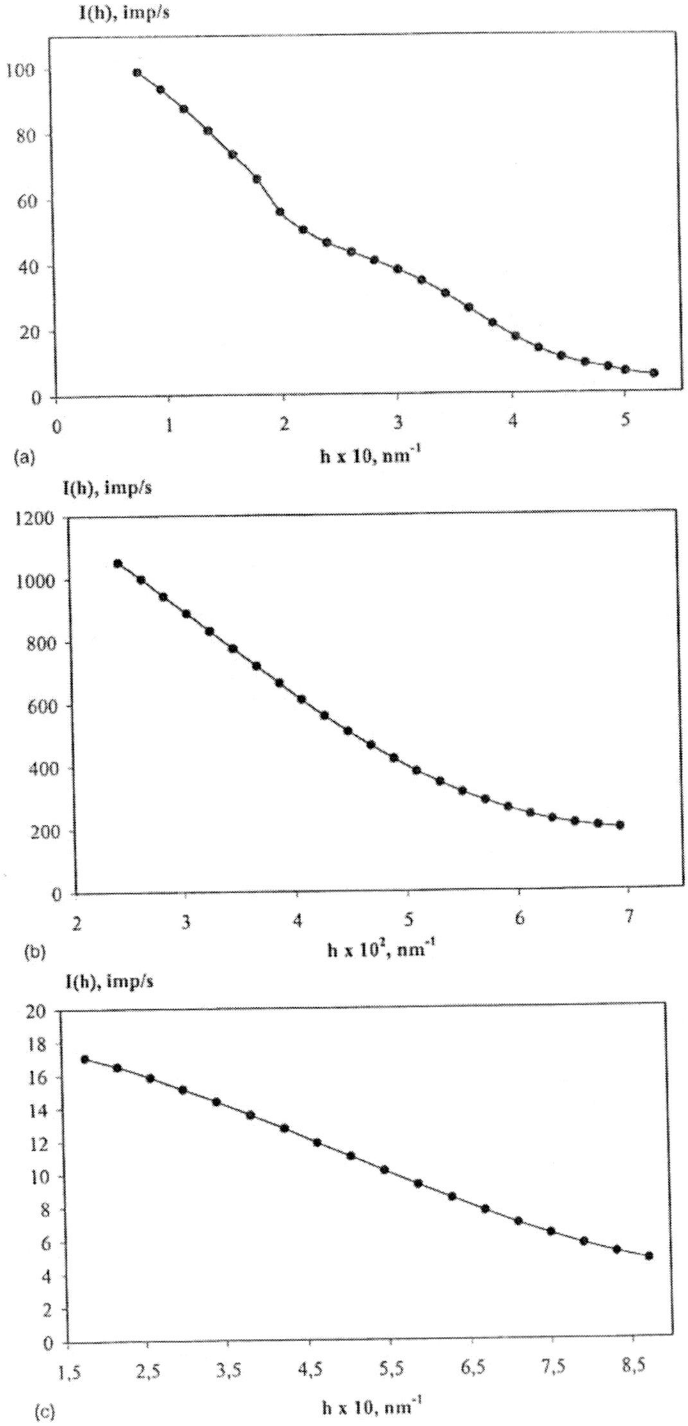

\Figure 7. SAXS plots of RNA-PM (a), DNA (b), and apoA-I (c) solutions in coordinates *I*(*h*), *h*. Concentrations of RNA-PM, apoA-I and DNA in solutions: 4.16, 0.3, and 3.12 mg/ml, respectively. With smoothing and corrections for background scattering and collimation of X-ray beam.

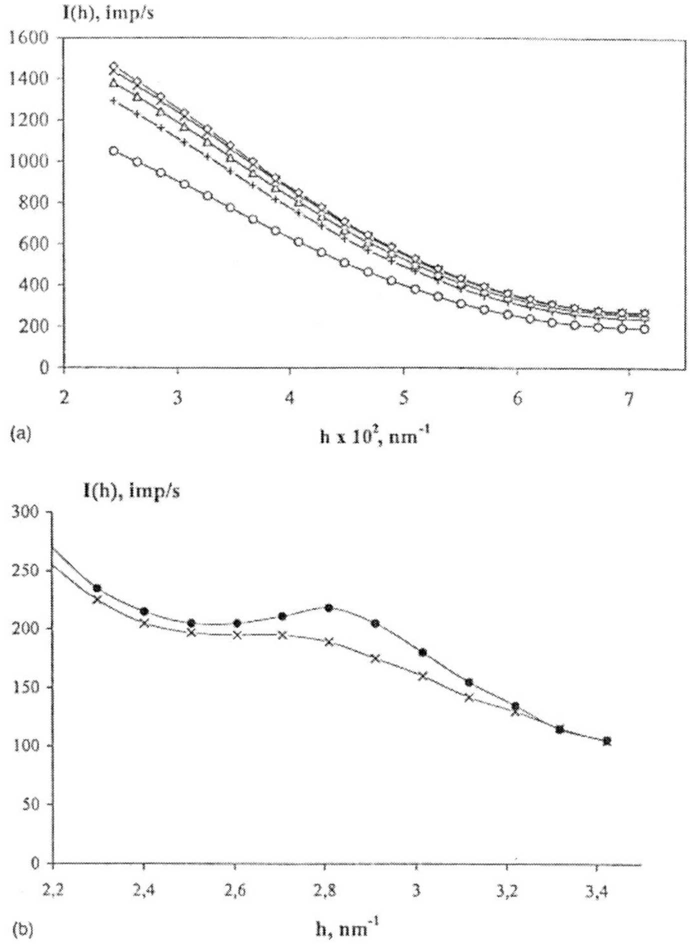

Figure 8. SAXS plots of solutions of free DNA (o) and four DNA mixtures with apoA-I and RNA-PM in the presence of THXC: (+) mixture 1; (Δ) mixture 2; (×) mixture 3; (◊) mixture 4 in the smallest angles (a) and in the region of diffraction peak at $h = 2.66$ nm^{-1} (b). Plots of the mixtures were taken at 37°C. DNA, RNA-PM, and apoA-I concentrations in mixtures 1-4 are shown in Table 12.

Such interaction resembles the enzyme–substrate interaction, in which hormone plays the role of a cofactor. The interaction results in the rupture of hydrogen bonds between the pairs of DNA nitrous bases and the formation of single-stranded structures.

To evaluate the stoichiometry of P*n*S complex formed due to RNA-PM (P) interaction with DNA-apoA-I-THC complex (S) we used a simplified scheme [43]:

$$n \cdot P + S \Leftrightarrow PnS , \qquad (2)$$

where n is the number of protein molecules bound into P*n*S complexes. From estimates obtained in our SAXS experiments (Table 12) and from the results of studies reported in [39, 40] one can assume that in these interactions the equilibrium is shifted essentially to the formation of complexes, i.e., it is highly cooperative.

Then, upon formation of P*n*S complexes in the mixtures, parameter n in scheme (2) will grow up to some maximum value with increasing protein concentration (C_p) in the mixtures. Using

(1) for estimation of the values of parameter n in each protein–DNA mixture, one can obtain the expression [43]:

$$n = M_s(T_{io} - 1)/M_p\,, \qquad (3)$$

where $T_{io} = (I_i(0)/I_o(0))^{1/2}$; $I_i(0)$ and $I_o(0)$ are the intensities of scattering to the zero angle (h = 0) from the i-mixture and initial DNA preparation, respectively.

In ref. [43] at the same component concentrations we obtained the value n for apoA-I upon complexation with DNA in the presence of THC equal to 54 ± 1. Table 12 presents the calculation results for parameter n and the estimates of Cp/Cs balance for all RNA-PM mixtures with DNA used in the study in the presence of THC-apoA-I complexes, taking $I_o(0)$ = 1605 imp/s. One can see that the n value in the mixtures does not exceed the values of the balance and in mixture 4 reaches its maximum at 6 ± 1. This corresponds to a 6:1 stoichiometry of the formed P*n*S complex.

In the above results, the sites of binding the THC-apoA-I complex to DNA remained unclear. Search for the supposed sequences over existing data bases revealed the presence of cis-element of $(GCC)_n$ type in the structure of human apoA-I gene.

It locates at the position of (+6) – (+16) nucleotide pairs from the translational stop-codon. Its position from the transcription starting point is (+896) – (+906) nucleotide pairs [43]. A similar sequence was revealed in the regulatory regions of many mammalian and human genes. It is quite conservative in terms of evolution and plays, probably, an important role in regulation of these genes expression and DNA replication.

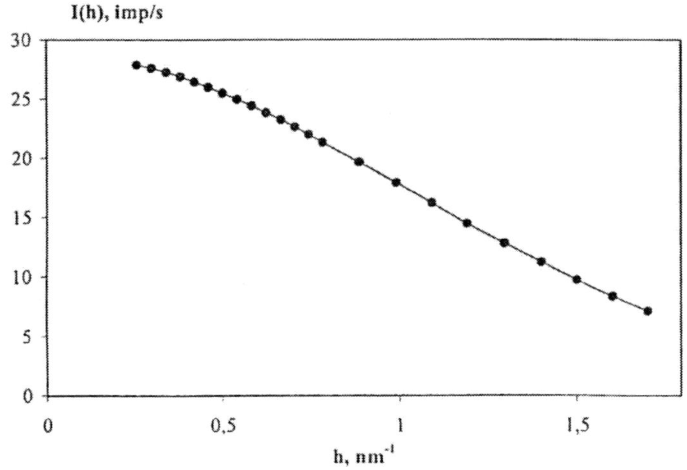

Figure 9. SAXS plot og oligonucleotide I solution in coordinates $I(h)$, h. Oligonucleotide concentration 1.52 mg/ml with corrections for background scattering and collimation of X-ray beam.

Further studies were performed with three synthetic oligonucleotides, whose structure was presented above (see Materials and methods). Figs. 7 and 9 show SAXS plots obtained from solutions of apoA-I (Fig. 7c) and oligonucleotide 1 (Fig. 9). Values of some structural characteristics of these macromolecules were calculated from the analysis of experimental data. ApoA-I molecules were shown to possess a slightly oblong shape with the ellipsoid axes ratio b/a = 3.6, radius of gyration Rg = 2.35 nm and molecular mass M = 27.4 kDa, which is close to the values we obtained earlier [43]. It is known that macromolecules of short single-chain oligonucleotides in a solution can have a common shape of the particles like ellipsoid of revolution or cylinder [19]. Thus, the values of radius of gyration (Rg = 1.2 ± 0.06 nm) and volume (V = 6.308 nm^3) we obtained for oligonucleotide 1 correspond to the structure of cylinder with 0.727 nm radius and 3.8 nm height.

To estimate by SAXS the effects of apoA-I interaction with oligonucleotides we used the equilibrium mixtures of oligonucleotides with apoA-I and its complexes with THC and cortisol. We prepared four main titration mixtures of apoA-I with oligonucleotide 1, two mixtures for estimating the effects of apoA-I interaction with oligonucleotides 2 and 3, and two mixtures for determining the THC and cortisol effect on apoA-I interaction with oligonucleotide 1. Average Rg values were calculated as well as differential intensities of scattering to the zero angle ($\Delta I(0)$) for all mixtures of apoA-I with oligonucleotides and steroids. Table 13 lists the values of calculated characteristics of the interaction, obtained from preparation apoA-I and its mixtures with oligonucleotides in the presence and in the absence of THC in the medium. One can see in Table 13 that substantial interaction of apoA-I was observed only with oligonucleotide 1. It should be noted that in the medium without THC or when it was substituted for cortisol, the effect of oligonucleotide 1 interaction with apoA-I was much lower as compared to the control mixture 2.

Table 13. Average values of radius of gyration (R_g), experimental ($\Delta I(0)$) and simulated ($\Delta J(0)$) differential intensities of X-ray scattering to the zero angle obtained from the SAXS data, at molar concentrations of protein (C_p) and oligonucleotide (C_s) in the mixtures

Mixture	Oligonucleotide	C_p (mkM)	C_s (mkM)	R_g (nm)	$\Delta I(0)$ (imp/s)	$\Delta J(0)$ (imp/s)
1	2	3	4	5	6	7
1	Oligo-1	6.6	51.5	2.25 ± 0.04	3.2 ± 0.3	3.16
2	Oligo-1	9.9	25.7	2.32 ± 0.05	2.9 ± 0.4	2.93
3	Oligo-1	11.3	14.3	2.35 ± 0.05	2.1 ± 0.2	2.06
4	Oligo-1	12.1	8.6	2.36 ± 0.05	1.1 ± 0.3	1.40
5	Oligo-2	9.9	25.7	2.35 ± 0.05	0.4 ± 0.3	-
6	Oligo-3	9.9	25.7	2.37 ± 0.05	0.3 ± 0.2	-
7[a]	Oligo-1	6.6	51.5	2.33 ± 0.05	1.5 ± 0.3	-
8[b]	Oligo-1	6.6	51.5	2.28 ± 0.04	1.1 ± 0.2	-

In mixture 1-6 THC is present witn concentration $2 \cdot 10^{-4}$ M. Primary structures of single-chain oligonucleotides: oligo-1 (oligonucleotide 1), oligo-2 (oligonucleotide 2), oligo-3 (oligonucleotide 3) are presented in Table column. 2.

[a] – In mixture 7 hormones are absent.

[b] – In mixture 8 cortisol is present with concentration $2 \cdot 10^{-4}$ M.

The changes of $\Delta I(0)$ value in mixtures 1–4 indicate that complexes of initial molecules form in the mixtures. The average size (Rg = 2.38 ± 0.07 nm) of $PmSn$ complexes (P are aggregates of apoA-I with THC; S is oligonucleotide; m, n are the number of protein and oligonucleotide molecules which bound into $PmSn$ complexes) is close to the size of apoA-I molecules in a free state, while the reliable changes were observed only in the values of $\Delta I(0)$ related to concentration and molecular mass of the complexes, similar to [43]; however, here $M = m \cdot Mp + n \cdot Ms$ (M is the molecular mass of $PmSn$ complexes involved into scattering).

To estimate the maximum stoichiometry of the complex formed as a result of interaction between oligonucleotide 1 (further oligonucleotide) and apoA-I we used the SAXS experimental data from the first four mixtures, the highly cooperative equilibrium scheme, and the methodology we developed earlier [39, 40]:

$$m \cdot \mathrm{P} + n \cdot \mathrm{S} \Leftrightarrow \mathrm{P}m\mathrm{S}n\ , \qquad (4)$$

$$K_{mn} = ([\mathrm{P}]^m \cdot [\mathrm{S}]^n) / [\mathrm{P}m\mathrm{S}n]\ ,$$

$$R(m, n, K_{mn}) = 2/p \cdot \Sigma\, |\Delta I_i(0) - \Delta J_i(0)| / (\Delta I_i(0) + \Delta J_i(0))\ ,$$

where K_{mn} is the dissociation constant for PmSn complex; [P], [S] and [PmSn] are the equilibrium concentrations of protein, oligonucleotide and complex, respectively; R is the optimization criterion; $\Delta I_i(0)$ and $\Delta J_i(0)$ are experimental and simulation values of differential intensities of scattering to the zero angle (h = 0). It follows from the data of Table 14 that the minimum value of R criterion corresponds to 1:1 stoichiometry of the formed complex (m = 1, n = 1) at the association constant (K_{ass}) = 1.66 · 10^6 M^{-1}. Using the $\Delta I_i(0)$ values obtained for mixtures 7–8 (see Table 13), we estimated the K_{ass} values for these mixtures, which appeared equal to 5.37 · 10^5 M^{-1} without THC in the mixture and 3.65 · 10^5 M^{-1} when THC was substituted for cortisol.

Table 14. Values of optimization criterion *R* (%) for the *m* × *n* matrix calculated from the SAXS experimental data

m	n		
	1	2	3
1	2.8 (K_{ass} = 1.66 · 10^6 M^{-1})	27.3	36.9
2	27.4	5.9	8.9
3	40.5	26.5	15.5

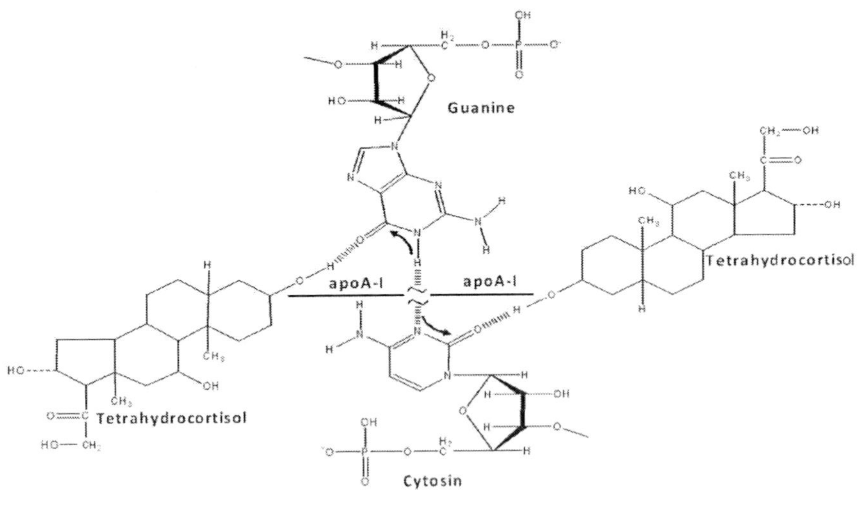

Figure 10. Schematic representation of the rupture mechanism of hydrogen bonds in GC-pairs of DNA under the action of THC – apoA-I complex.

Molecular mechanisms of the interaction of hormone-apoA-I complex with DNA are illustrated by an example with THC. Two molecules of the hormone are shown to be involved in the interaction with GC pairs of DNA (Fig. 10). OH group of the first molecule concurrently splits the left hydrogen bond, and that of the second molecule splits the right hydrogen bond in GC pair. This leads to redistribution of electron density in the internal hydrogen bond and its cleavage. Local melting of DNA occurs, which increases due to hydrophobic interaction between nitrogen base rings and hydrophobic regions of α-helices of apoA-I. This mechanism was verified by IR spectroscopy study [46].

3.5. Contribution of Macrophages to the Mechanism of Intracellular Regeneration of Various Organs and Tissues

ApoA-I as a transport form delivering steroid hormones to the cell nuclei was determined in the fraction of acidic nonhistone proteins. This fraction includes a large number of proteins responsible for the regulation of gene expression. The fraction under consideration was obtained from the cell nuclei of brain, liver, kidneys, lungs, heart, skeletal muscles, adrenal glands, testicles, spleen, and red bone marrow. The study was performed using the Dot analysis. ApoA-I immunoreactivity was detected in the cell nuclei of all organs and tissues. The immunoreactivity was most pronounced in the nuclei of red bone marrow, spleen and liver. These organs exhibit the highest functional and proliferative activity. The lowest level of immunoreactivity was observed in skeletal muscles. Other organs showed the intermediate values (Fig. 11).

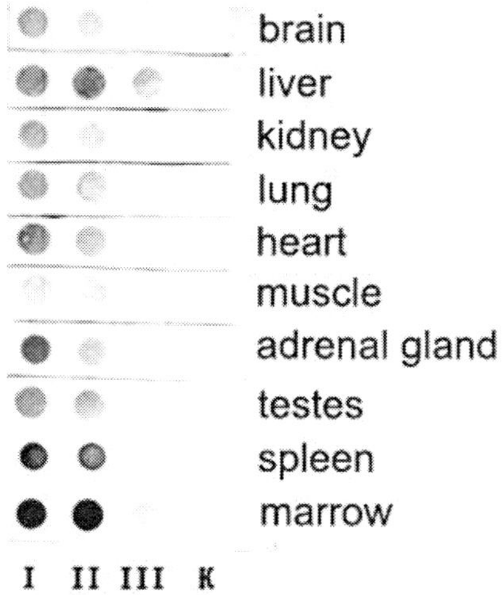

Figure 11. Dot-analysis of apoA-I immunoreactivity in nuclear fractions of various rat tissues. I, II, III – dilutions 1:1, 1:2, 1:10. K – control.

The obtained results are important not only in terms of the regulation of gene expression with participation of hormone – apoA-I complex, but also with respect to delivery of various lipids (cholesterol, phospholipids, and antioxidants) to the cell nuclei.

Lipids are the constituting elements of chromatin and nuclear membrane, they play an important role not only in their structural, but also functional organization. In this connection, of great interest is the fact revealed in our study: cell nuclei of some organs contain not only apoA-I, but also apoB and apoE [47]. ApoB was represented by the products of its limited proteolysis. Electrophoresis and subsequent immunoblotting make it possible to detect 6-8 fractions with apoB immunoreactivity. All three apolipoproteins interact with lipids and are considered as their essential transport species [37].

The contribution of macrophages to the mechanisms of intracellular regeneration in various organs and tissues was estimated from the rate of ^{14}C leucine incorporation into total protein. Macrophages were stimulated with LPS, which were injected intravenously 24 h before the injection of ^{14}C leucine. The latter was injected intraperitoneally. In these experiments, we failed to obtain complete reproducibility of results.

A positive stimulating response was observed usually in the liver, kidneys, spleen, thymus, and red bone marrow. Unstable data were obtained for the lungs, heart, skeletal muscles, and brain. However, repeated experiments allowed us to observe the enhancement of protein biosynthesis in these organs at in vivo stimulation of macrophages. In one of experiments, an increase in protein biosynthesis rate attained 25% in brain, 47% in heart, and 64% in muscles. The rates of protein biosynthesis expressed in radioactivity units were equal, respectively, to (6.6±0.4, 6.6±0.4, 5.3±0.3) $\cdot 10^2$ imp/min per mg protein in the control; and (8.3±0.7, 9.7±0.7, 8.8±1.6)$\cdot 10^2$ imp/min per mg protein in the experiment. Three days after LPS stimulation of macrophages, high rate of protein biosynthesis was observed only in the red bone marrow. In the brain, skeletal muscles, adrenal glands, thymus and spleen, a reliable difference from the control was not found. In the liver, kidneys, lungs and brain, the rate was reliably lower.

It seems that in each experiment the animals form a certain priority of the organs that are able to enhance protein biosynthesis in response to LPS stimulation of macrophages. This priority may change with experiments. However, a positive response can be obtained virtually in all tissues (Fig. 12).

It remains unclear whether the enhancement of protein biosynthesis in different organs is produced by LPS stimulation of all resident macrophages or this is the stimulation of only the most accessible pool - Kupffer cells in hepatic sinusoids. The second assumption seems more likely, because activation occurs mainly in Kupffer cells. These are the cells where the biologically active complex THC-apoA-I is formed; it readily penetrates through histohematogenous barrier in various organs and initiates protein synthesis. However, it is not clear which additional conditions can facilitate the operation of this mechanism. Analysis of this issue requires further investigation.

Conclusion

Macrophages are polyfunctional cells. They are present in all organs and tissues without exception. Their common source is represented by hemopoietic stem cell of the bone marrow, which goes through several stages of differentiation: monoblast → promonocyte → bone marrow monocyte → peripheral blood monocyte → tissue macrophage. Differentiation of this cell terminates in the tissues, where it transforms into the tissue-specific (resident) macrophage. Of tremendous importance for the organism is the liver pool of macrophages — Kupffer cells. They reside on the internal surface of hepatic sinusoid and contact directly the flowing blood. This allows them to perform a very important clearing function in the organism. However, through fenestations of the endothelial lining, macrophages migrate to the liver beams where they come into contact with hepatocytes. This underlies the involvement of macrophages in numerous metabolic relations. Together with hepatocytes, they take part in the metabolism of lipoproteins, steroid hormones, hemoglobin, etc.

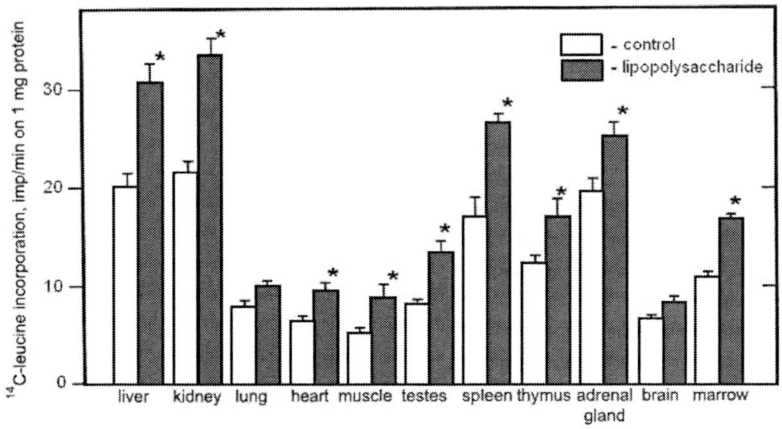

Figure 12. Change in the rate of protein biosynthesis in the rat organs and tissue 24 hours after injection of bacterial LPS. * - significant changes relative to control.

In case of necessity, macrophages can move completely into the liver interstitial space to participate in regeneration of parenchymal cells. To date, this extremely important role of macrophages is studied insufficiently.

Partial liver resection according to Higgins and Anderson, i.e., the removal of 2/3 of the organ weight, is a convenient model for investigation of this function of macrophages. Great research attention is focused now on implementation of various genetic programs. It is elucidatedc which genes are most active in different phases of regeneration: earlier [48], later [49], and terminal ones [50]. The contribution of cytokines and various growth factors to the regeneration mechanism is also explored [51]. However, little attention is paid to molecular mechanisms of intercellular interactions in the dynamics of liver regeneration after PLR [52]. This concerns particularly the interactions in the system "macrophage – parenchymal cell". Such studies were performed earlier [2]; however, no further development was made.

The fact that cell regeneration rate depends on the activity of macrophages is indisputable now. We have shown that stimulation of macrophages with LPS increases the mitotic activity of hepatocytes and shifts it to the earlier periods. On the contrary, loading of macrophages with Indian ink or colloidal iron decreases the maximum of mitotic activity and shifts it to the later periods (Fig. 3).

The role of macrophages in regeneration mechanisms can hardly be overstressed. It is known that macrophages activated by different methods (products of cell degradation, LPS, bacteria, foreign particles, etc.) secrete a large amount of biologically active compounds into the internal medium [2, 36]. Among them are lysosomal enzymes (collagenase, elastase, lysozyme, β-glucuronidase, cathepsins, etc.), monokines, and factors of natural resistance (interferons, complement proteins, etc.). These compounds help the dividing cells to overcome contact inhibition.

A great contribution to regeneration is made not only by lysosomal enzymes of macrophages, but also by the own lysosomes of dividing cells, in which free activity of lysosomal enzymes is increased. Our studies showed that HDL can increase both the free activity of lysosomal proteases and translocations of lysosomes to the nucleus [34]. This leads to destruction of the nuclear membrane and deproteinization of DNA (see Fig. 4 and Table 4).

This is the first work demonstrating an important role of different class lipoproteins in cell regeneration. It was found that synthesis and secretion of VLDL and LDL are induced in a regenerating liver. The dividing cells need building materials. This may be a reason for raising the blood content of VLDL and LDL, which can be used as a source of phospholipids and cholesterol in the formation of biological cell membranes. An increased antioxidant protection plays a notable role here. Blood lipoproteins are known to provide transport of tocopherols to the cells [27].

HDL and steroid hormones (glucocorticoids) play a special role in cell regeneration. PLR is followed by cooperative capture of HDL_3 and glucocorticoids by Kupffer cells. Their stimulation with LPS enhances the cooperative capture mechanism.

An action of HDL on chromosomal DNA from the different tissue and cells attracts considerable attention of researches. At present, the mitogen-stimulating function of HDL is widely discussed in the literature. The stimulating effect of HDL was demonstrated for the proliferation of lymphocytes [53], epithelial [54], endothelial [55], smooth muscle [56], and tumor [57] cells. It is known that in the G_1-period of mitotic cycle the mRNA and protein synthesis increases, in the S-period the mRNA, rRNA and protein synthesis increases, in the G_2-period the mRNA, rRNA and protein synthesis proceeds and proteins-initiators are formed, in the M-period proteins-initiators are activated and DNA is reduplicated. In the absence of protein synthesis the cells cannot pass the mitosis stage and enter the next mitotic cycle. The causes of these cell changes in premitotic period are still not clear.

Structural analysis of the genes presented in International banks (GenBank, EMBL DNA library) revealed the presence of recurrent $(GCC)_n$. These recurrences are found in both prokaryotic and eukaryotic genes, in human genes as well. The number of such recurrences varies and may be very great. Such recurrences ("packets") stabilize the DNA structure, at the same time they hamper its reduplication. They imply a special mechanism favoring the rupture of hydrogen bonds in such "packets". Our studies allow to conclude that the formation of THC-apoA-I complex may serve as such mechanism. It leads to a complete separation of complementary strands of DNA and the subsequent doubling it with the participation of DNA polymerase.

Formation of this complex is related to the resident macrophages, which control the intracellular regeneration and proliferation of cells. They possess a remarkable ability to restore double bonds in A ring of steroid hormones yielding tetrahydrocompounds. This process is catalyzed by α- and β-reductases [58]. Our studies showed that tetrahydrocortisol and other steroid hormones form the biologically active complex with apoA-I enhancing the synthesis of DNA, RNA, and protein [43]. In this case, apolipoprotein A-I acts as a targeted carrier to the cells nuclei. This complex is formed in macrophages. The source of apoA-I are HDL, which are cooperatively captured by macrophages together with the products of cells degradation [59].

Thus, for the first time in the present work a specific interaction of THC-apoA-I complex with eukaryotic DNA and the kinetics of this interaction were described, structural characteristics of apoA-I, oligonucleotide $CC(GCC)_5$, and their complexes in the presence of cortisol and THC were determined. It was assumed that THC-apoA-I complexes interact with DNA regions containing $(GCC)_n$ elements, which results in the rupture of hydrogen bonds between the pairs of DNA nitrous bases. Partially untressed sections of DNA double chain are the targets for RNA-PM, whose binding and functioning are greatly affected by local denaturation of DNA and formation of single-stranded regions [60], though it is known that RNA-PM can bind also to the native DNA. It was shown for the first time that the reduced forms of glucocorticoids, tetrahydrocompounds, are the biologically active form of hormone involved in the enhancement of gene expression, entering the composition of THC-apoA-I complex. In this case, apoA-I acts as a targeted carrier, and reduced form of hormone favors the rupture of hydrogen bonds between the pairs of DNA nitrous bases, causing its local denaturation and creating prerequisites for interaction as RNA-PM as DNA-polymerase with single-stranded DNA regions. The described mechanism is schematically shown in Fig. 10. Macrophages play a key role in its formation.

References

[1] Wakabayashi G, Shimazu M, Ueda M, Tanabe M, Kawachi S, Kitajima M. Liver regeneration after resection: molecular and cellular mechanism. *Nihon Geka Gakkai Zasshi*. 2004; 105 (10): 650-653.

[2] Mayansky D, Wisse E, Decker K. New Frontiers of hepatology. *Nauka*, Novosibirsk, 1992.

[3] Xu W, Wang S, Wang G, Wei H, He F, Yang X. Identification and characterization of differentially expressed genes in the early response phase during liver regeneration. *Biochem Biophys. Res. Commun*. 2000; 278 (2): 318-325.

[4] Zimmermann A. Regulation of liver regeneration. *Nephrol. Dial. Transplant*. 2004; Suppl. 4: 6-10.

[5] Fujiyoshi M, Ozaki M. Molecular mechanisms of liver regeneration and protection for treatment of liver dysfunction and diseases. *J. Hepatobiliary Pancreat. Sci.*. 2011; 18 (1); 13-22.

[6] Kountouras J, Boura P, Lygidakis NJ. Liver regeneration after hepatectomy. *Hepatogastroenterology*. 2001; 48 (38): 556-562.

[7] Ross MA, Sander CM, Kleeb TB, Watkins SC, Stolz DB. Spatiotemporal expression of angiogenesis growth factor receptors during the revascularization of regenerating rat liver. *Hepatology*. 2001; 34 (6): 1135-1148.

[8] Terui K, Ozaki M. The role of STAT3 in liver regeneration. *Drugs Today (Barc)*. 2005; 41 (7): 461-469.

[9] Gnainsky Y, Spira G, Paizi M, Bruck R, Nagler A, Genina O, Taub R, Halevy O, Pines M. Involvement of the tyrosine phosphatase early gene of liver regeneration (PRL-1) in cell cycle and in liver regeneration and fibrosis effect of halofuginone. *Cell Tissue Res*. 2006; 324 (30): 385-394.

[10] Tang W, Liang K, Wang J, Du L, Zhang W. Effects of pHGF on hepatocyte DNA synthesis after partial hepatectomy in rats. *J. Tongji Med. Univ.* 1998; 18 (1): 25-27.

[11] Nadal C. Dose-related opposite effects of hydrocortisone on hepatocyte proliferation in the rat. *Liver*. 1995; 15 (2): 63-69.

[12] Kutsyĭ MP, Zakrzhevskaia DT, Gaziev AI. Hydrocortisone and partial hepatectomy activate a proteinase associated with histones. *Biokhimiia*. 1992; 57 (10): 1548-1553.

[13] Schmid W, Sekeris CE. Nucleolar RNA synthesis in the liver of partially hepatectomized and cortisol-treated rats. *Biochim Biophys Acta*. 1975; 402 (2): 244-252.

[14] Panin LE, Kunitsyn VG, Tusikov FV. *Effect of glucocorticoids and their complexes with apolipoprotein A-I on the secondary structure of eukaryotic DNA. Intern. J. Quantum Chem.* 2005; 101 (4): 450-467.

[15] Panin LE. Molecular mechanisms of interaction of THC - apoA-I complex with DNA and initiation of transcription. In: Corly R. Woods. editor. Trends in DNA research. Nova Science Publishers Inc; 2006. p. 65-102.

[16] Li CJ, Li RW, Elsasser TH. Alpha-tocopherol modulates transcriptional activities that affect essential biological processes in bovine cells. *Gene Regul. Syst. Bio*. 2010; 22 (4): 109-124.

[17] Chocian G, Zabielski P, Chabowski A. Liver regeneration after partial hepatectomy. Role of lipid mediators. *Postepy Hig Med Dosw*. 2002; 56 (1): 49-71.

[18] Lenz M, Miehe WP, Vahrenwald F, Bruchelt G, Schweizer P, Girgert R. Cholesterol based antineoplastic strategies. *Anticancer Res*. 1997; 17 (2A): 1143-1146.

[19] *Higgins GM, Anderson RM*. Experimental pathology of the liver: Restoration of the liver of the white rat following partial removal. *Arch. Pathol.* 1931; 12: 186–202.

[20] Pokrovskii AA, Archakov AI, Methods of separation and identification of subcellular fractions of the enzymes. In: *Modern methods in biochemistry*. Meditsina, Moscow. 1968. pp.5-59.

[21] Barrett AJ. Lysosomal enzymes. In: Lysosomes, A Laboratory Handbook. North-Holland Pub Co., Amsterdam; 1972. pp 46–136.

[22] Lowry OH, Rosebrough N.J, Farr AL, Randall RJ. Protein measurement with the Folin phenol reagent. *J. Biol. Chem.* 1951; 193 (1): 265-275.

[23] Pankov YA, Usvatova IJ. Fluorometric method for determination of 11-hydroxycorticosteroids in peripheral blood plasma. In: *Methods for determination of certain hormones and neurotransmitters*. Moscow; 1965. pp. 137-145.

[24] Laemmli UK. Cleavage of structural proteins during the assembly of the head of bacteriophage T4. *Nature*. 1970; 227: 680-685.

[25] Szego CM. Lysosomal function in nucleocytoplasmic communication. *Front Biol.* 1975; 43 (4): 385-477.

[26] Vladimirov YA, Dobretsov GE. *Fluorescent probes to study biological membranes.* Nauka, Moscow; 1980. 320 p.

[27] Panin LE, Polyakov LM, Kolosova NG, Russkikh GS, Poteryaeva ON. Distribution of tocopherol and apolipoprotein A-I-immunoreactivity in rat liver chromatin. *Biol. Membranes*. 1998; 11 (5): 631-640.

[28] Panin LE, Tuzikov FV, Tuzikova NA, Polyakov LM. Features of interaction of complexes cortisol-apolipoprotein A-I and tetrahydrocortisol- apolipoprotein A-I with eucariotic DNA. *Mol. Biol. (Mosk).* 2006: 40 (2): 300-309. Russian.

[29] Panin LE., Maksimov VF, Usynin IF, Korostyshevskaya IM. Activation of nucleolar DNA expression in hepatocytes by glucocorticoids and high density lipoproteins. *J. Steroid Biochem. Mol. Biol.* 2002; 81 (1): 69-76.

[30] Fraker PJ, Speck JC. Protein and cell membrane iodinations with a sparingly soluble chloroamide, 1,3,4,6-tetrachloro-3a, 6a-diphenylglycosuril. *Biochem. Biophys. Res. Commun.* 1978; 80 (4): 849-857.

[31] Fatyol K, Illes K, Diamond DC, Janish C, Szalay AA. Mer22-related sequence elements form pericentric repetitive DNA families in primates. *Mol. Gen. Genet.* 2000; 262 (6): 931-939.

[32] Grant CE, Kurz EU, Cole SP, Deeley RG. Analysis of the intron-exon organization of the human multidrug-resistance protein gene (MRP) and alternative splicing of its mRNA. *Genomics.* 1997; 45 (2): 368-378.

[33] Kunitsyn VG, Panin LE, Polyakov LM. Anomalous change of viscosity and conductivity in Blood plasma lipoprotein in the physiological temperature. *Intern. J. Quantum Chem.* 2001; 81 (5): 348-369.

[34] Panin LE, Mayanskaya NN. *Lysosomes: their role in adaptation and recovery.* Nauka, Novosibirsk; 1987. 198 p.

[35] Panin LE. *Stress, heart and blood vessels. In: Problems of atherosclerosis.* SB RAMS, Novosibirsk; 2005. pp. 20-34.

[36] Mayansky DN. Lectures on Clinical Pathology: manual. *GEOTAR Media,* Moscow; 2008. 464 p.

[37] Klimov AN, Niculcheva NG. *Exchange of lipids and lipoproteins and its disorders.* Peter Com, St. Petersburg; 1999. 512p.

[38] Hoschenko OM. *Biochemical mechanisms of participation of resident macrophages in the regulation of the biosynthesis of DNA and protein in normal and tumor cells of the liver.* Thesis, Novosibirsk; 2002.

[39] Tuzikov FV, Zinoviev VV, Vavilin VI, Maligin EG, Ankilova VN, Moor NA, Lavrik OI. Application of the small-angle X-ray scattering technique for the study of equilibrium enzyme-substrate interactions of phenylalanyl-tRNA synthetase from E. coli with tRNAPhe. *FEBS Lett.* 1988; 232 (1): 107-110.

[40] Tuzikov FV, Zinoviev VV, Vavilin VI, Malygin EG. Application of the small-angle X-ray scattering technique for the study of two-step equilibrium enzyme-substrate interactions. *Biopolymers.* 1996; 38 (2): 131-139.

[41] Tuzikov FV, Panin LE, Tuzikova NA, Polyakov LM. Application of the small-angle X-ray scattering technique for estimating structural changes in high density lipoproteins. *Membr. and Cell Biol.* 1996; 10 (1): 75-82.

[42] Stöckel P, May R, Strell I, Cejka Z, Hoppe W, Heumann H, Zillig W, Crespi H. The core subunit structure in RNA polymerase holoenzyme determined by neutron small-angle scattering. *Eur. J. Biochem.* 1980; 112 (2): 411-417.

[43] Panin LE, Tuzikov FV, Tuzikova NA, Khar'kovskiĭ AV, Usynin IF. Effect of tetrahydrocortisol-apolipoprotein A-I complex on protein biosynthesis in hepatocytes and secondary structure of eukaryotic DNA. *Mol. Biol. (Moskow).* 1999; 33 (4): 673-678.

[44] Svergun DI, Feigin LA. In: X-ray and neutron small-angle scattering. Nauka, Moscow (Russian); 1986. p.279.

[45] Watson D. Molecular Biology of the Gene. Mir, Moscow; 1978. pp. 281-412.

[46] Panin LE, Kunitsyn VG. The initiation mechanisms of gene expression in ascitic hepatoma cells under the action of dehydroepiandrosterone in a complex with apolipoprotein A-I. *J. Current Chemical Biology*. 2009; 3 (3): 306-314.

[47] Panin LE, Russkikh GS, Polyakov LM. Detection of apolipoprotein A-I, B and E immunoreactivity in the nuclei of various rat tissue cells. *Biochemistry* (Mosc). 2000; 65 (12): 1419-1423.

[48] Juskeviciute E, Vadigepalli R, Hoek JB. Temporal and functional profile of the transcriptional regulatory network in the early regenerative response to partial hepatectomy in the rat. *BMC Genomics*. 2008; 9: 527-532.

[49] Kountouras J, Boura P, Lygidakis NJ. Liver regeneration after hepatectomy. *Hepatogastroenterology*. 2001; 48 (38): 556-562.

[50] Fausto N. Liver regeneration. *J. Hepatology*. 2000; 32 (1 Suppl.): 19-31.

[51] Fausto N, Campbell JS, Riehle K.J. Liver regeneration. *J. Hepatology*. 2006; 43 (2 Suppl 1): 45-53.

[52] Michalopoulos GK, DeFrances M. Liver regeneration. *Adv. Biochem. Eng. Biotechnol.* 2005; 93: 101-134.

[53] Favre G, Blancy E, Tournier JF, Soula G. Proliferative effect of high density lipoprotein (HDL) and HDL fractions ($HDL_{1,2}$, HDL_3) on virus transformed lymphoblastoid cells. *Biochim. Biophys. Acta*. 1989; 1013 (2): 118-124.

[54] Biran S, Horowitz AT, Fuks Z, Vlodavsky I. High-density lipoprotein and extracellular matrix promotes growth and plating efficiency of normal human mammary epithelial cells in serum-free medium. *Int. J. Cancer.* 1983; 31 (5): 557-566.

[55] Tamagaki T, Sawada S, Imamura H, Tada Y, Yamasaki S, Toratani A, Sato T, Komatsu S, Akamatsu N, Yamagami M, Kobayashi K, Kato K, Yamamoto K, Shirai K, Yamada K, Higaki T, Nakagawa K, Tsuji H, Nakagawa M. Effects of high-density lipoproteins on intracellular pH and proliferation of human vascular endothelial cells. *Atherosclerosis*. 1996; 123: 73-82.

[56] Resink TJ, Bochkov VN., Hahn AW, Philippova MP, Bühler FR, Tkachuk VA. Low- and high-density lipoproteins as mitogenic factors for vascular smooth muscle cells: individual, additive and synergistic effects. *J. Vasc. Res.* 1995; 32 (5): 328-338.

[57] Favre G, Tazi KA, Le Gaillard F, Bennis F, Hachem H, Soula G. High density lipoprotein3 binding sites are related to DNA biosynthesis in the adenocarcinoma cell line A549. *J. Lipid Res.* 1993; 34 (7): 1093-1106.

[58] Sawyer NJ, Oliver JT, Troop RS. Observation on the role of the RES in the metabolism of adrenocortical steroids. *Steroids*. 1963; 2: 213-227.

[59] Panin LE. Phenomen of stimulation protein biosynthesis in parenchymal cells of organs and tissues by resident macrophages. *Bull. SB RAMS* (Russian). 1998; 3: 11-23.

[60] Panin LE, Gimautdinova OI, Poliakov LM, Naiakshina TN. Characteristics of interaction of cortisol, tetrahydrocortisol, and their complexes with apolipoprotein A-I with eukaryotic DNA. *Mol. Biol.* (Moskow). 1998; 32 (3): 447-451.

In: Apolipoproteins
Editors: A. D. Sidorov and M. Y. Nikitin
ISBN: 978-1-62257-484-1

Chapter II

Current Concepts on the Formation of Discoidal Apolipoprotein A-I Lipid Bound Complexes: From Picket Fences to a Double-Belt Model via Inter-Ring Rotation of Apolipoprotein A-I Monomers

Thomas R. Caulfield[*]
Department of Neuroscience, Mayo Clinic Florida,
Jacksonville, Florida, US

Abstract

The double belt model for lipid-bound discoidal apolipoprotein A-I consists of two alpha-helical monomers bound about an unilamellar bilayer of lipids. Previous work, based on salt bridge calculations, has demonstrated that the L5/5 registration, Milano mutant, and Paris mutant are preferred conformations for apolipoprotein A-I. Additional recent research has indicated that there is a possibility of inter-ring rotation between the two monomers about the lipid unilamellar bilayer core. For instance, from well-known mutations, the Paris (R151C) and Milano (R173C) mutants indicate a mode of change must be available. To find proper registration, one proposed change is a 'rotationally' independent circular motion of the two protein monomers about the lipid unilamellar bilayer core. Current research shows that from a computational perspective, the independent inter-ring rotation of the two alpha-helical monomers about the lipid unilamellar bilayer core is feasible. And, such simulations support the existing double-belt model. Other long time scale dynamics simulations are very revealing of the discoidal behavior having preferred out-of-plane shapes akin to a saddle-point. However, despite all of the indicated deformations, the rotation of the two protein monomers is able

[*] Correspondence: Thomas R Caulfield, Ph.D. Telephone: 404-275-3684, Fax: 904-953-2449. E-mail: caulfield.thomas@mayo.edu.

to occur with biasing. It was determined that a cysteine mutant at Glu107 as a possible target for future mutational studies. Several other biophysical studies are discussed in light of these recent findings to bring a greater understanding to ApoA-I dynamic motion and registration shifts. Since HDL remodeling is necessary for cholesterol transport, our model for remodeling through dynamics has substantial biomedical implications.

Keywords: Apolipoprotein A-I, discoidal high density lipoprotein, HDL, double belt model, Paris mutant, Milano mutant, simulation

I. Introduction

Apolipoprotein-AI (Apo A-I) has a demonstrated vital role among the cholesterol maintenance mechanisms available in mammals [1]. Antiatherogenic high-density lipoprotein (HDL) contains ApoA-I as a key component. ApoA-I is comprised as a supramolecular assembly composed of protein monomers associated with other lipophilic molecules, like phospholipids and cholesterol), which for example includes HDL [2, 3]. Reverse transport of cholesterol from tissues to the liver for elimination are promoted via the efflux from tissues where ApoA-I and the lecithin cholesterol acyltransferase (LCAT) participate. ApoA-I, a key component of plasma HDL, is found in chylomicrons. ApoA-I is synthesized in liver cells and small intestine cells [4, 5]. Important lipid transport and cholesterol recycling processes are important for biosynthesizing new molecules, maintainence of cellular functioning in mammals, and reduced risk of atherosclerosis [6-8]. Additionally, ApoA-I is found as a constituent of spheroidal and discoidal nascent HDL particles.

I.1. The Structural Arrangement for Apolipoprotein A-I Discoidal Pucks, Competing Models Picket-Fence and Double-Belt

Numerous models for ApoA-I have been discussed in the literature [9-11]. Molecular modeling has greatly helped improved the understanding of structural biomechanisms, and refinement of the model with further experiments. The double belt model, which has been previously noted in the literature, as an attractive basis for remodeling [9].

Presented here is recent work on the Apo A-I double belt model that originated from the lab of Dr. Stephen C. Harvery and Dr. Jere Segrest. The original double belt model consisted of two basic protein sequences, which run in antiparallel directions with overall alpha-helical orientation punctuated with histindine hinge-points. N-terminus domain for Apo A-I contains residues 1 through 43. The c-terminal domain, lipid binding domain, contains residues 44 to 243, and 44 to 247 for other models. The structure for the N-terminal domain is considered to be globular in some cases, and helical in others, however more recent experimental work has used AFM and CD to determine a random-coil with mostly globular structure. These fragments of Apo A-I were obtained in a lipid free environment, whilst a helical state is found in lipid-mimicking detergent [12].

Another competing model for the discoidal HDL has been described thoroughly in the literature [9-11]. For this model, the double belt model contains 160 lipids appropriated into a small unilamellar bilayer [9]. The assembly of the two protein chains forms circular rings around a collection of lipids. The belt's structure contains two ampipathic α-helix protein chains. Apo A-I's α-helix forms 3.67 residues per turn, contains a hydrophobic surface facing the lipids, and has an optimal geometry to form intermolecular salt bridge interactions with an antiparallel arrangement that matches the lipid free crystal structure [13]. Each protein α-helix contains eight 22-mer and two 11-mer tandem amino acid sequence repeats. The periodicities of the two monomers of ApoA-I are punctuated by prolines, which aid in maintaining the circular geometry [14]. Previous work supports a preference for the double belt model, but is still debated [15]. Non-specific hydrophobic interactions, inter-helical salt bridges, and a mode of dynamic electrostatic movement that allows the specificity of helix-helix registration drive Apo A-I binding in the discoidal HDL particle. Previously, the belt model using molecular dynamics and HDL and POPC lipids supported inter-helical registration with the use of a helical wheel. Some molecular dynamics experiments have profiled lipid behavior under varying conditions [17]. Inter-helical salt bridges determine the preference for one antiparallel interface and dictate the registration of the helices [18-21], where the maximal salt bridging model corresponded to the alignment found in the apo Δ(1-43) A-I crystal structure [13]. More recent work has probed extensively the dynamic motion underpinning the requirements to form the orientations, or remodeled complexes, required for the mutant forms to occur from the native conformation generated in-silico [16].

I.2. Disease Specific Mutants of ApoA-I (Paris and Milan) Point to Double-Belt Model for Remodeling Complexes

Several interesting diseases involve mutations of the ApoA-I native sequence. In particular, a mutation occurs with the arginine to cysteine mutants. For different population groups, the mutation is in different points of the sequence. The two populations mentioned here, originated from Milan and Paris. The milan mutation of apoA-I_{Milano} is residue 173, while the Paris mutation is residue 151 [22-24]. Moreover, wild-type ApoA-I lacks the cysteine residues in the genetic sequence [22]. Of interest, either the Arg to Cys mutation does not adversely affect the reconstituted mutant HDL particles. Also, both the mutant HDL particles and the *wt* HDL particles are equally capable of clearing dimyristoyl-phosphatidyl-choline (DMPC) emulsions and promote normal cholesterol efflux [25-27]. Populations with the Paris and Milano mutation have shown decreased levels of HDL, yet paradoxically, also a reduced risk for atherosclerosis [22, 23, 26].

ApoA-I_{Milano} reconstitutes into HDL particles, with either two or four distinct molecules of apoA-I, forming in two diameters. Reconstituted HDL particles have a size similar to wild-type ApoA-I HDL particles [24, 25]. Yet apoA-I_{Paris} HDL particles form into particles with three possible diameters [28].

Differing helical registrations exist for the models of ApoA-I, and were examined interaction energies between the helix-helix side chains of the two protein monomers of the double belt model [29]. More recently the author has shown dynamic movement for reorganization of the helical registration is possible and presents complex interaction energies [16]. Prior to this recent work, it was hypothesized a mode of re-assigning the registrations was possible, allowing shifts between registrations after the discoidal complex forms. Current experimental work on the mechanism for different registrations forming is on going. The

Milano and Paris-type mutants have shown that ApoA-I forms a disulfide bond between the cysteine residues, thus locking the protein monomers fixed in that static conformation. Yet, if different registrations of Paris and Milano variants were to form after initial synthesis, mobility of the protein monomers would be necessary to associate under alternate registrations.

Derived from the original belt model for ApoA-I and the Paris and Milano in the literature [15, 24], the author has simulated a new models for the independent rotation of the two protein monomers. Derived from *wt* apoA-I, the author constructed a molecular dynamics simulation over a 360° rotation of the two monomers [16]. Exploring each registration along this path, the interaction energy was plotted, revealing an inherent stability in the Paris and Milano mutants from salt bridge interactions [16]. The author defined four other low energy states, three of which are lower in energy than the Paris and Milano mutants [16]. The methods section below recapitulates the novelty in the model and technique [16].

II. Methods Used in Modeling the Dynamic Motion of the Double Belt Models

The intial state for the belt model for ApoA-I was formerly published [14, 15]. The model generated therein was carried out with INSIGHT and the Quanta package on an SGI workstation [30]. The author's modeling described throughout was completed using VMD for molecular setup [31]. Simulations were determined using NAMD [32, 33] and scripting languages to alter NAMD MD-engine parameters (force vectors, etc). The author utilized the well-known and previously published models from the Harvey and Segrest Labs [29, 34-37]. The author's study acts as a launch point for future studies on heterodimers and different orientations [16].

II.1. Revisiting the Methods in Detail from the MdMD Method for Biasing

Each simulation system consisted of a periodic box containing the Apolipoprotein A-I protein, 176 molecules of POPC lipids in a bilayer, and solvent molecules, for a total of ~165, 000 atoms.

We added two Na+ counterions to neutralize the simulation cell, and then added sufficient Na+ and Cl- ions replicating a physiological solution. In the random initial placement of ions, a minimum distance of 10 Å between the ions was maintained, and the ions were placed in bulk water and away from the protein. A typical simulation cell is visible in the supplemental materials (Movie S1). The apoA-I protein plus POPC lipid bilayer was fully solvated using TIP3P water molecules in a box of dimensions 164 x 160 x 115 $Å^3$ [38]. The periodic cells were designed that the minimum distance between the molecules and the edge of the water box was 20 Å. Our results indicate that the ApoA-I and POPC residues do not interact with the edge at edge-to-edge distances > 35 Å, thus we expect the size of the cell is sufficient to prevent interaction between molecules in neighboring cells. Two Na+ ions were added to balance the charge of the terminal protein residues, and then sodium and chloride ions were added, yielding electric neutrality in the unit cells. Simulations were run using a constant number of particle, volume, and temperature conditions and all used periodic boundary conditions. Simulations were run in NAMD using the CHARMM27 parameter set with a timestep of 2 fs using SHAKE [32, 39, 40]. Electrostatics interactions were calculated using the particle-mesh Ewald method [41]. Nonbonded interactions had a real-space cutoff of 15 Å. The systems were minimized 4000 steps of steepest decent with the apo A-I/POPC complex held fixed, then subsequently, for an additional 4000 steps of the adopted-basis Newton-Raphson method with decreasing harmonic restraints on the apo A-I/POPC complex. Each system was then equilibrated for 100 ps with the apo A-I/POPC complex fixed with a harmonic restraint of 0.5 kcal/mol applied to the heavy atoms of ApoA-I and POPC, so that only solvent and ions were free to move. Each system was then equilibrated for another 150 ps with the temperature coupling to a heat bath of 310 K under constant volume conditions with gradually relaxing restraints, 0.5 kcal/mol/Å^2 to 0.25 kcal/mol/Å^2 to 0.13 kcal/mol/Å^2 (50 ps each), and then under constant volume conditions with no restraints for 100 ps [42, 43]. The simulation temperature was kept constant using the Berendsen algorithm by weakly (τ_p = 0.1 ps) coupling the protein, lipid, and solvent to a temperature bath of 310 K [44]. Likewise, the pressure was kept constant by isotropically coupling the system to a pressure bath of 1 bar, with a coupling constant of τ_p = 2 ps and a compressibility of 4.5 x 10^{-5} bar $^{-1}$. Restrained equilibration runs were done for 5 ns to ensure the system stability, while low restraint k < 1kcal/mol was applied at Cα atoms to maintain the original starting structure for production runs under Maxwell's demon molecular dynamics (MdMD) runs [45]. MdMD has been previously described in the literture [45]. Here we present the use of the MdMD method for sampling rare conformational pathways by removing entropy from the system (Figure S2). Table 1 outlines the various MdMD schemes used for sampling with MD intervals called *MDsprints*. Figure 7 shows a schematic for the MdMD algorithm, which has been previously discussed [45].

Briefly, the MdMD method repeated scans a direction of conformations using short intervals of MD called "MDsprints", where at the end of each sprint the "demon" measures the system for a global property, in this case, the relative position of the two protein monomers along the Z-axis, such that we are aiming for z-angle increasing for each monomer relative to the other. The MDsprint may be anywhere from 50 femtoseconds to 10 picoseconds. If the measure property has satisfied the Maxwellian demon (score) with an incremental increase, decrease, or other measurable property, like the amount of rotation measured relative to the two protein monomers, then the MDsprint is maintained in an archive file, whilst if the sprint is a failure, then it is annulled and the system restarts from the last archived state. From the last archived state, the system may be reinitialized for velocities upon the waters (stp) derived from a Boltzman distribution of the system. This is a "randomizer" for the Mdsprints. Total simulation time amongst all runs, including disregarded states of sampling, would be > 1 microsecond of MD sampling. However, the archived success states for all conformations that move incrementally forward based on the biasing scheme totals approximately 100 ns. In the case of parallel motion between the two protein monomers, successful rotations were completed in 3 nanoseconds of MdMD, which corresponds to over 300 ns of total MD time with a 1 percent success rate. Likewise, for the 30 nanosecond rotations achieved using MdMD, over 800 ns of MD time with 2-4 percent success rate on each run. In all simulations that utilized our Maxwell's demon biasing algorithm [46], a structure from the previous state's run was used to start each successive run.

Coordinates were saved between 2 and 40 ps intervals. Biasing forces are applied with a constant force of 20 pN as shown in Figure 2. This force is only applied as a projection onto the X-Y plane relative to the Z-axis of rotation, which is defined by the center of the ApoA-I protein monomers ring-like structure. This force is applied at n and n+7 Cα atoms. Additionally, the constant force-biasing algorithm may be coupled with all other atoms to sample conformational space during the course of the simulation.

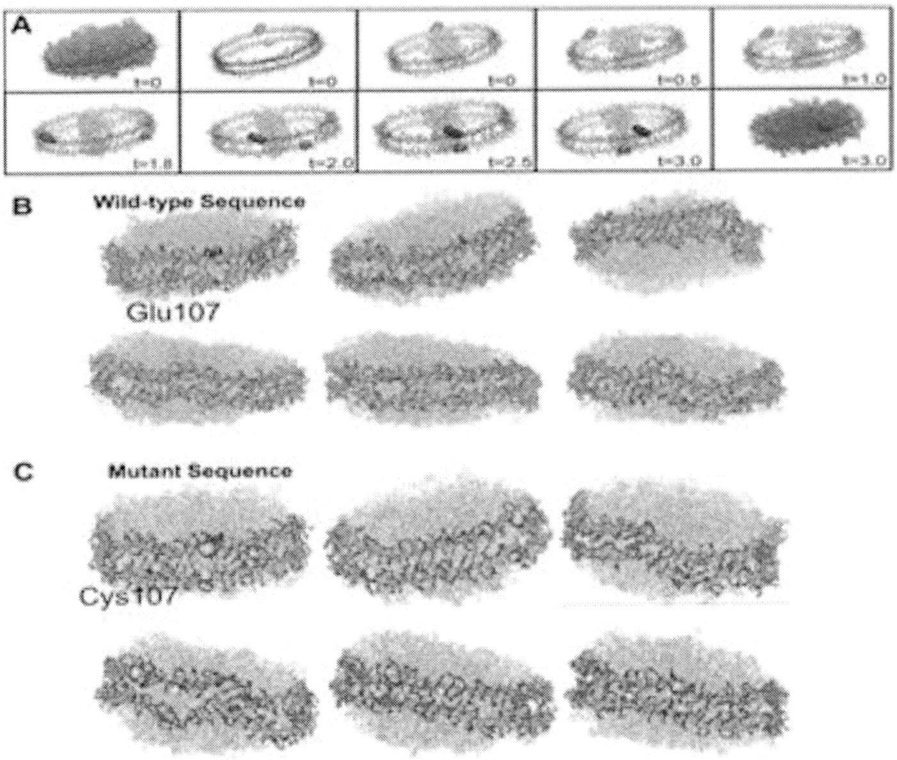

Figure 1. Discoidal ApoA-I HDL particle inter-ring rotation using biased MdMD. A. Idealized rotation of Apolipoprotein A-I driven along a circular path in X-Y plane, using by a biasing Tcl-forces script using namd2. This circular path is invoked with a 40pN force vector pointed between the Cα_n and Cα_{n+7} atoms in the X-Y plane. The initial three panel shows t=0ns, where the lipids are only removed visually to allow for easier viewing. Lipids (176 POPC residues) are present during entire 3ns. In the third panel on top, two ampipathic α-helical ApoA-I monomers (in red and blue) are rendered in licorice, while a small core of lipids (in yellow) illustrates overall stability during simulation. Using VdW rendering, enlarged residues (red and blue) clearly show the initial position of the two rings. The VdW residues highlight the pathway. B. Non-idealized rotation of native sequence for Apolipoprotein A-I driven using by a biasing with MdMD Tcl-forces algorithm implemented in namd2. This circular path is invoked with a 20pN net force vector between Cα_n and Cα_{n+7} pairs. Which is projected onto the X-Y plane. A slow application of MdMD is applied biasing the sampling time. Non-perfect planarity of the protein monomers is achieved, while rotation continues as in the idealized case Figure 1A. Steps along the trajectory are shown with arrows separating different times in the pathway. C. Non-idealized rotation of mutant (Glu107Cys) sequence for Apolipoprotein A-I driven using by a biasing with MdMD Tcl-forces algorithm implemented in namd2. This circular path is invoked with a 20pN net force vector between Cα_n and Cα_{n+7} pairs. Which is projected onto the X-Y plane. A slow application of MdMD is applied biasing the sampling time. Non-perfect planarity of the protein monomers is achieved, while rotation continues as in the idealized case Figure 1A. Steps along the trajectory are shown with arrows separating different times in the pathway.

Table 1. Summary of MdMD Simulations for apolipoprotein-AI

Structure Name	apoAI native (3ns MdMD sampling)	apoAI mutant (3ns MdMD samping)	apoAI native (25-30ns MdMD sampling)	apoAI mutant (25-30ns MdMD sampling)
Structure Source	Initial model coordinates (Klon et al., 2006 and Harvey/Segrest personal communication)	Initial model coordinates (Klon et al., 2006 and Harvey/Segrest personal communication)	Initial model coordinates (Klon et al., 2006 and Harvey/Segrest personal communication)	Initial model coordinates (Klon et al., 2006 and Harvey/Segrest personal communication)
Protein residue range	α: 1-203	α: 1-203	α: 1-203	α: 1-203
Metal ions in protein	Physiological Na+, Cl- concentration	Physiological Na+, Cl- concentration	Physiological Na+, Cl- concentration	Physiological Na+, Cl- concentration
Number of runs	3	2	1	1
Equilibration water box size	164×160×114 Å^3	164×160×114 Å^3	164×160×114 Å^3	164×160×114 Å^3
Correct step per no. incorrect steps (overall % success; MdMD rate)	1% (percent retained from total sampling of all *MDsprints*)	1% (percent retained from total sampling of all *MDsprints*)	2-3% (percent retained from total sampling of all *MDsprints*)	2-3% (percent retained from total sampling of all *MDsprints*)
Number of atoms for equilibration	149,167 to 151,033	149,167 to 151,033	149,167 to 151,033	149,167 to 151,033
Specialized TCL-forces applied during simulations	3 constant-force applied runs totaling ~300 ns sampling time with 1% success rate with force applied from C_n to C_{n+7} direction in X-Y plane	2 constant-force applied runs totaling ~300 ns sampling time with 1% success rate with force applied from C_n to C_{n+7} direction in X-Y plane	2 constant-force applied runs totaling ~800 ns sampling time with 3% success rate with force applied from C_n to C_{n+7} direction in X-Y plane	1 constant-force applied runs totaling ~800 ns sampling time with 3% success rate with force applied from C_n to C_{n+7} direction in X-Y plane
Total sampling time from every MD sprint (both archived and abandoned samples)	3 MdMD totaling ~900 ns sampling	2 MdMD totaling ~600 ns sampling	1 MdMD totaling ~800 ns sampling	1 MdMD totaling ~800 ns sampling

With the subset of biasing on Cα's, we utilized an iterative and adaptive algorithm called Maxwell's demon (MdMD) (Movie S2). MdMD utilizes intervals of MD ranging from 50 fs to 10 ps in duration.

After each interval, a global variable is measured, measuring parameters of the system. This method has been previously reported [46]. MdMD was done with a size-optimizing search for the best time-length interval for optimal sampling (Figure 2).

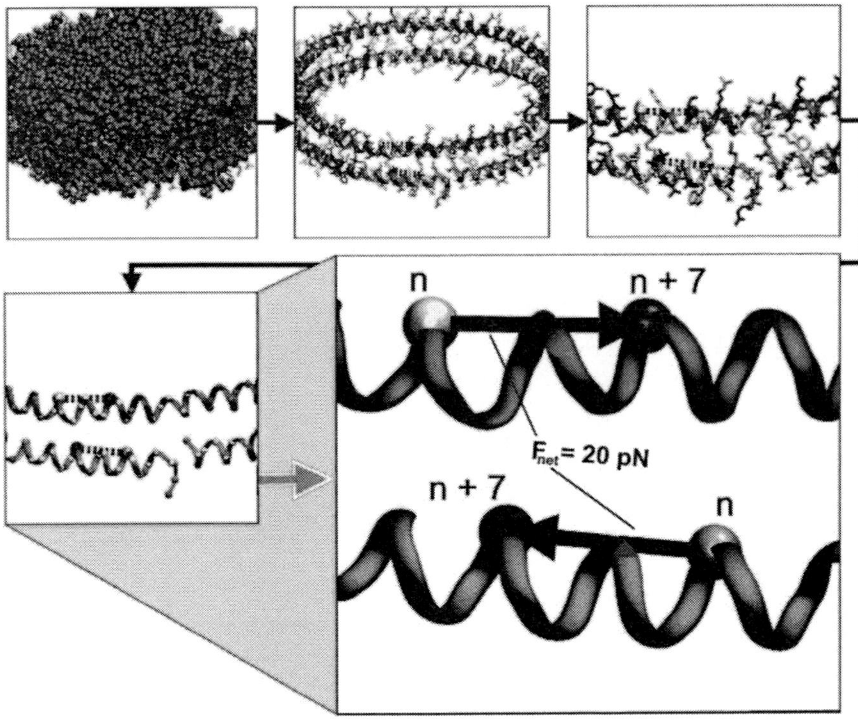

Figure 2. Biasing Scheme. Schematic for the Apolipoprotein-AI Tcl-Forces. Shown above on the left is the apolipoprotein-AI complex. The two protein ring monomers are colored red and blue to easily distinguish between them. The side chains are shown in licorice with a rainbow color scheme to distinguish residues. In the second panel, the lipids are not shown to reveal the shape of the two ring monomers. The third panel zooms in to reveal the alpha-helical shape and the interacting side chains. A dotted line shows the vector path of the force applied between n and n+7. The next panel simplifies this showing only Cα atoms and the alpha helix shape as a tube. The last panel zooms on two example pairs. The vectors applied to the two monomers A and B, the ampipathic α-helical proteins, are in opposite direction. The individual example force vector shown, F=10pN per C-alpha pair, is projected from the XYZ direction between n and n+7 onto the X-Y plane, which uses a 20pN net force on both pairs above, or 10pN per Calpha pair. Additional information on the MdMD biasing scheme is in Supplemental Figure S2.

The biggest limitation to any MdMD study is the length of time for desired transition to occur. In the longer MdMD simulations (30 ns runs), we lowered our TCL-forces applied from C_n to C_{n+7}, which were mapped onto the XY-plane (to remove any Z-axis unraveling). The criterion for success was made more lenient to allow for larger MDsprints (time between scoring up to 10ps) before assessing with the demon. For both the mutant (Glu107Cys) and native sequence, the 3-nanosecond MdMD run archive (contains all of the cumulative successes), a non-planar, non-idealized model results. The structure for the apolipoprotein from MdMD more closely matches the shapes described in the literature [47]. However, bear in mind the 3-nanoseconds cumalitive-MdMD run is approximately 300-nanoseconds of conformational landscape sampled in the direction of the reaction coordinate that results in a 180° rotation of apolipoprotein monomer 1 (ring 1) relative to apolipoprotein monomer 2 (ring 2). Likewise, there is a 180° rotation for ring 2 relative to ring 1 occurs, thus giving the appearance of 360° rotation. Supplemental Table 1 contains the specific details of simulations. Additionally, we did native and mutant simulations for very slow rotational sampling with a net result of around 25-30 nanosconds of successful MDsprints, which corresponds to over 800 ns of sampling time. A mutation of Glu107 to Cys107 was modeling in using the VMD plugin [31]. Results from the Glu107 energy profile (see results) indicated testing Cys107 for indicated mutational studies. As described above, minimization, equilibration, production and MdMD biasing were conducted on the mutant to achieve similar results. Both a short run and a long MdMD biasing run were conducted on the Glu107Cys mutant.

III. A Discussion of the Current Understanding of the Inter-Ring Rotation of the Double Belt Model via MD Biasing

III.1. Rotation of the Monomer Rings of ApoA-I is Possible with a Biasing Potential

The author found evidence supporting independent inter-ring rotation of the two alpha-helical monomers about the unilamellar bilayer contained within the core [16]. The protein monomers successfully moved in a 'forward' anti-parallel direction is using MdMD biasing (Supplemental Movie S1 and Movie S2). Additionally, biasing forces were applied (see scheme (20 pN per n, n+7 Cα) shown in Figure 2). Whereas, the time for the forward direction occurs in approximately 3 ns (of MdMD time), the reverse direction requires approximately 4.5 ns (of MdMD time) and has more disorder in inter-protein side chain interactions.

III.2. 'Ring Rotation' Has an Independent Feature

Figure 1A shows a continuous series of snapshots based on the idealized simulation of the discoidal ApoA-I protein/POPC lipid complex (3.4 ns MdMD run time). In the series of snapshots the time (as indicated in the lower left corner). At frame 1 time = 0ns, we can see a detailed molecular belt model for apolipoprotein A-I. In frame 2 time = 0ns, the lipids (gray) was removed (only graphically removed) to show both protein monomers of ApoA-I (red and blue). As well, two large VdW representations of residues are shown, indicating motion. In frame 3 time = 0ns, a core lipids (yellow) are visually reintroduced to illustrate the relative stability of lipids during simulations. In frame 4 time = 0.5ns, the initial motion of the two monomers is shown. In frame 5 time = 1.0ns to frame 9 time = 3.0ns, we see the movement of the two rings about the Z-axis. Lastly, in frame 10, time = 3.0ns, the lipids are redrawn to show any conformational change. Supplemental Movie S1 shows the idealized ring rotation.

Figure 1B is a continuous series of snapshots from both the native sequence and mutant sequence of the discoidal ApoA-I protein/POPC lipid complex (3.4 ns MdMD run time). A series of snapshots reveals the global conformational changes and 360° ring rotation as indicated by the reference molecule shown on each monomer as a large green sphere. The native sequence simulation has the same sequence as the ApoA-I in Figure 1A. However, in this case the amount of MdMD sampling time in the interval between examinations was increased from 60 fs to 600 fs and the force applied with the TCL-forces from each C_n to C_{n+7}

(mapped onto the XY-plane) was lowered from the original 40 pN per pair to 20 pN per pair. These lowered parameters define our non-idealized system. In the case of POPC lipid bound ApoA-I discoidal complex under these conditions has distortion from the planarity of the idealized model in Figure 1A. Figure 1B shows many conformational states observed in other thermal based MD studies and long-run dynamics simulations [36, 37, 47, 48]. Interesting conformers were analyzed for energies from the entire archived trajectory (Figure 5A). The mutant sequence has lower interaction energy between the two monomers at the Gly89/Ser188 and Glu107Cys mutation. The Gly88/Ser188 was not tested for a mutation simulation, but may bear repeating. The Glu107Cys mutation (purple line—Figure 5A) is approximately 1kcal/mol lower than in the native sequence (black line—Figure 5A) at 2.5 ns MdMD run time. However, we note that there is also a lowered energy for the mutant at the Paris position around 1 ns of MdMD run time.

Figure 1C is a continuous series of snapshots from both the native sequence and the mutant sequence of the discoidal ApoA-I protein/POPC lipid complex (25 ns MdMD run time). A series of snapshots reveals the global conformational changes and 360° ring rotation as indicated by the reference molecule shown on each monomer as a large green sphere. The native sequence simulation has the same sequence as the ApoA-I in Figure 1A. However, in this case the amount of MdMD sampling time in the interval between examinations was increased between 100 fs to 5000 fs and the force applied with the TCL-forces from each C_n to C_{n+7} (mapped onto the XY-plane) was lowered from the original 40 pN per pair to 20 pN per pair. These lowered parameters define our non-idealized system. In the case of POPC lipid bound ApoA-I discoidal complex under these conditions has significant distortions from the planarity of the idealized model in Figure 1A. Figure 1C shows several conformational states observed in other thermal based MD studies and long-run dynamics simulations [36, 37, 47, 48]. Interesting conformers were analyzed for energies from the entire archived trajectory (Figure 5B).

Figure 5C shows the mutant sequence has nominally lower interaction energy at the two monomers of the Gly89/Ser188 orientation. However, the mutant versus the native is nearly within twice the standard deviation, 0.256, at Gly or Ser188. However, the Milano paired conformation is significantly lower for the mutant than for the native sequence at a time of 4 ns MdMD run time. And the Paris position is worse for the mutant than the native sequence at a time of 7-8 ns of MdMD run time. Even more, the mutant is poor scoring for the Tyr126 paired orientation versus the native sequence with a different in interaction energy of over 2 kcal/mol. Figure 5B shows the Glu107 position is lower for the mutant but within the standard deviation for the longer amount of 23 ns MdMD run time. Supplemental Movie S2 and Movie S3 detail the MdMD-derived rotational motion for these systems.

It must be emphasized that a simulation of 3 nanoseconds with MdMD is not equivalent to 3 nanoseconds of MD. MdMD is only archiving successful steps as measured by the Maxwellian demon (Figure S2). Incorrect, or bad steps, are discarded. With a success rate between 1% and 4%, and in some simulations under 1%, the total sampling time is large. For ring rotation of 3 ns, the true sampling time is approximately 300 ns. Slower rotational rate, with lower force, yields better success rates.

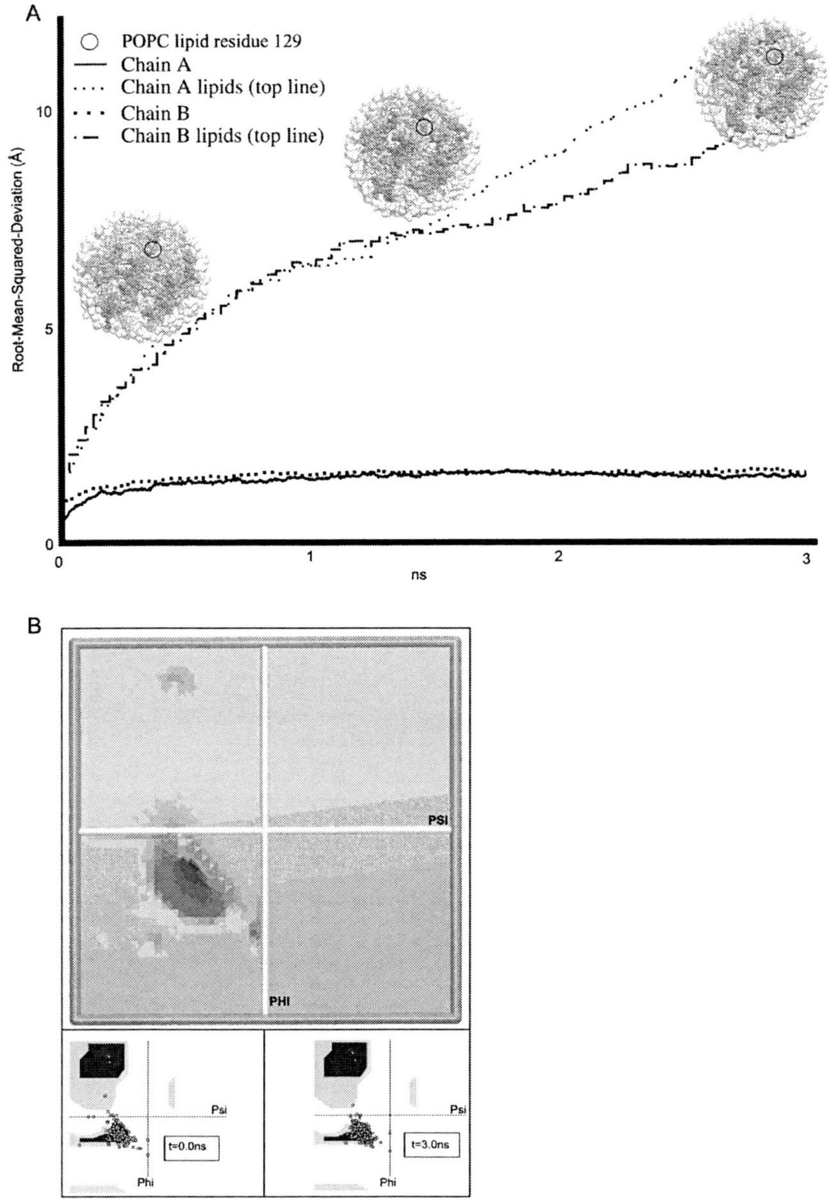

Figure 3. RMSD and PHI/PSI Plot. RMSD for the two molecules of the ampipathic α-helical ApoA-I monomers and the Phi/Psi space that the protein chains A and B during 3ns simulation. A. RMSD of ~2Å for the two protein chains is show at the bottom of the graph. Shown in dotted and dot-dashed line above is the lipid RMSD for the 3ns simulation. The unconfined lipid is free to move about; both lipid tails and headgroups RMSD grows from 3 to 10Å. However, the overall POPC lipids are not deformed. The black circle shows the migration of POPC residue 129, which is fairly stable over the entire 3ns trajectory. B. Phi/Psi plots for the apolipoprotein-AI protein complex. The two protein ring monomers are shown in the contour map to illustrate the dominant α-helical character. The lower two Phi/Psi plots illustrate the α-helical character at the start and finish of the simulation. The two outliers on the upper left quadrant are the N- and C-terminal residues.

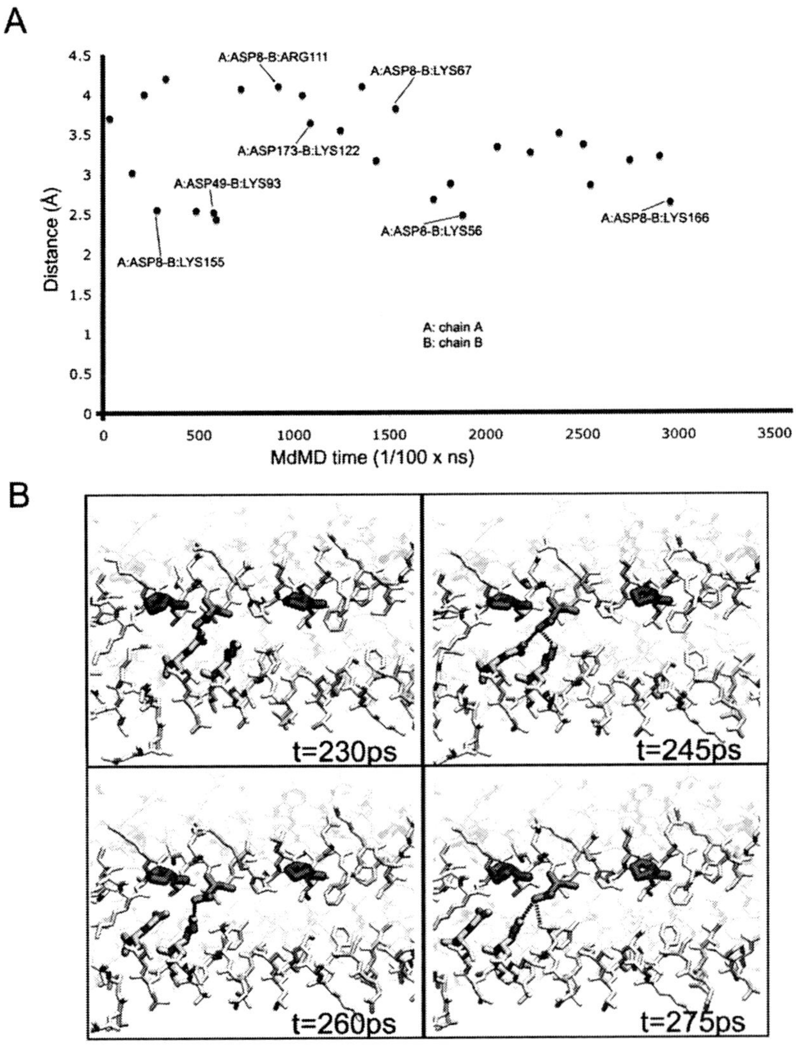

Figure 4. Salt Walking, H-bond Walking and Representative Salt Bridge Interactions. The ampipathic α-helical apo A-I protein monomers (chain A and B) undergo a 360° rotation during the course of the 3.5 ns simulation. Over the course of this simulation time, intermolecular interactions form and break between chain A and chain B >165 times and between chain B and chain A >169 times. Salt bridges and hydrogen bond pairs formed in the side chain pairs between the two monomers formed and lost during the course of the simulation is >340. A salt bridge is defined as a distance-based interaction between the oxygen atom of the acidic residue and the nitrogen atom of the basic residue. The avg. length of the salt bridge was 3.35Å with 95% of the salt bridges occurring between 2.77Å and 3.93Å. Bridges that formed between acidic monomers of chain A: ASP8, ASP49, ASP173, GLU30, GLU38, GLU45, GLU52, GLU70, GLU71, GLU85, GLU96, GLU107, GLU129, GLU143, GLU151, GLU158, GLU195 and basic monomers of chain B: ARG111, ARG133, ARG137, ARG151, ARG173, HSP115, HSP122, HSP159, LYS5, LYS19, LYS56, LYS67, LYS78, LYS93, LYS100, LYS155, LYS166, LYS199, and bridges formed between acidic monomers of chain B: ASP8, ASP49, ASP173, GLU30, GLU38, GLU45, GLU52, GLU70, GLU71, GLU85, GLU96, GLU107, GLU129, GLU143, GLU151, GLU158, GLU195 and basic monomers of chain A: ARG111, ARG133, ARG137, ARG151, ARG173, HSP115, HSP122, HSP159, LYS5, LYS19, LYS56, LYS67, LYS78, LYS93, LYS100, LYS155, LYS166, LYS199.

III.3. The Effect of Using MdMD for Biasing the Rotation of the Monomer Rings of ApoA-I

A schematic for the ApoA-I biasing method using Tcl-forces is shown in Figure 2. In the top left panel the original apolipoprotein-AI complex (protein—red and blue, lipids—gray). The model uses an α11/3 helical ring dimer that circumscribes an inner diameter of 85Å and outer diameter of 105Å. The 85Å diameter patch consists of a 176 POPC bilayer. The second panel shows only the two protein ring monomers (red and blue) to reveal the shape of the two ring monomers. The side chains are shown in licorice (spectrum color scheme). The third panel zooms in to reveal the alpha-helical shape and the interacting side chains. A series of dotted lines in panel 3 show the approximate vector path for the force vector applied between residue n and residue n+7. The fourth panel simplifies the rendering by only showing the Cα atoms that are affected by the biasing force (α-helix shape shown as tubes). The fifth panel zooms on an example pair. The tcl-force biasing vector is visualized. The vector is applied to both of the two ampipathic α-helical ApoA-I monomers A and B, but in opposite direction. The bottom monomer illustrates the force vector (F = 20pN), which is projected from the XYZ coordinates between n and n+7 onto an X-Y plane defined at the center of the ApoA-I rings. The direction of the force applied is always in the n to n+7 direction with a force of 20 pN. For 203 residues, there are 29 force vectors for all Cα atom in an XY plane. The amount of force was determined in an exhaustive series of simulations. Lower force resulted in unappreciable change in rotation, while larger forces derailed the monomer from the lipid bilayer (Supplemental Movie S3).

III.4. Implications for HDL Structure as a Result from the Remodeled Complexes Found in Molecular Dynamics

Figure 3 depicts an analysis of the stability of the protein monomer-monomer *rings* and lipids during the 3 ns simulation for the idealized system shown in Figure 1A. Figure3A shows the ampipathic α-helical ApoA-I monomers A and B are within 2.5 Å of their original conformation for the 3ns simulation. This result abides well the biasing force with the required α-helical parameters required. Figure3B shows the top Phi-Psi plot places the α-helical parameters within the desired region. The large peak represents the sum of all Phi-Psi in that region. The average $\phi = -58°$ and average $\varphi = -49°$, which is consistent with an α11/3 helix. The two outliers we found at approximately (-60°, 75°) were due to the N-terminus (1) and C-terminus (203) residue having a freer range of motion. The Phi-Psi plot at the bottom of Figure 3B shows both the initial (t=0ns) and final conformation (t=3ns), indicating a stable protein structure throughout the simulation. Figure 3A shows where the lipids have much more conformational searching. The POPC lipids range from 3 Å to around 10 Å RMSD over the 3ns simulation. However, following one residue, POPC129 (shown in black circle), we observe that the relative position within the bilayer is unchanged. It has freedom to explore conformational space, but maintains position during simulation. Similar distributions for the Phi-Psi space were found amongst all models.

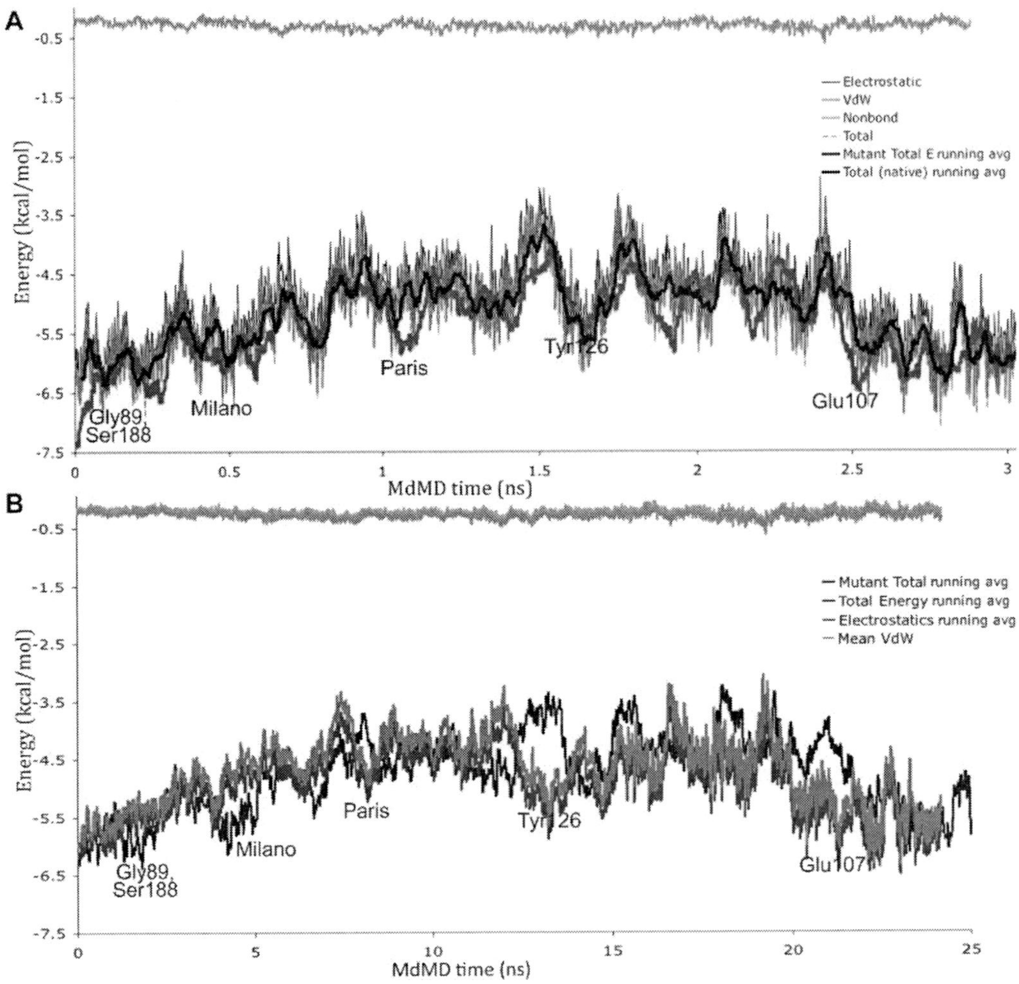

Figure 5. Energies of stable conformers. Interaction energies for the two protein monomers of the ampipathic α-helical ApoA-I calculated over 3 ns of MdMD run time (300 ns sample time) and 30 ns MdMD run time (~800 ns sample time). .A. The graph illustrates the energy output for the 3 ns MdMD run time, corresponding to ~300 ns of MD sampling time. The Paris (R173C) and Milano (R151C) mutation locations occur at time = 0.5 ns MdMD run time and 1.2 ns MdMD run time, respectively. Tyr126 exhibits similar energetic properties at time = 1.72 ns. Improved energetic conformations were observed at Ser184 (t=0.15 ns MdMD run time), Glu107 (t=2.52 ns MdMD run time). The energies spread over all 406 residues amongst the two monomers of 203 apiece, accounts for around 4.5 and 7.5 kcal/mol, slightly above the nominal thermal barriers. B. The graph illustrates the energy output of the 25 ns MdMD run time, corresponding to ~800 ns of MD sampling time. The Paris (R173C) and Milano (R151C) mutation locations occur at time = 5 ns MdMD run time and 8.5 ns MdMD run time, respectively. Tyr126 exhibits similar energetic properties at time = 14.5 ns. Improved energetic conformations were observed at Ser184 (t=2.0 ns MdMD run time), Glu107 (t=21 ns MdMD run time). The energies spread over all 406 residues amongst the two monomers of 203 apiece, accounts for around 4.5 and 6.5 kcal/mol, slightly above the nominal thermal barriers.

III.5. Interactions between the Two Protein Monomers during Rotation Intervals

We measure all salt bridge interactions between acidic and basic residues from monomer A to monomer B and from monomer B to monomer A during the 3ns simulation. We defined the criterion for the formation of a salt bridge when the interaction distance between the oxygen atoms of acidic residues and the nitrogen atoms of basic residues are within an average cut-off distance of 3.2 Angstroms over the course of the trajectory timeline. The overall average salt bridge distance was found to be 3.35 Å with a standard deviation of 0.58. As measured by distance, 67% of measured salt bridges were within 2.77Å and 3.39Å. From protein monomer A to B, 165 salt bridges were formed and broken, while from protein monomer B to A, 169 salt bridges were formed and broken during the 3ns simulation. A total of 334 salt bridges were formed and lost during the simulation.

Bridges that formed between acidic monomers of chain A: ASP8, ASP49, ASP173, GLU30, GLU38, GLU45, GLU52, GLU70, GLU71, GLU85, GLU96, GLU107, GLU129, GLU143, GLU151, GLU158, GLU195 and basic monomers of chain B: ARG111, ARG133, ARG137, ARG151, ARG173, HSP115, HSP122, HSP159, LYS5, LYS19, LYS56, LYS67, LYS78, LYS93, LYS100, LYS155, LYS166, LYS199, and bridges formed between acidic monomers of chain B: ASP8, ASP49, ASP173, GLU30, GLU38, GLU45, GLU52, GLU70, GLU71, GLU85, GLU96, GLU107, GLU129, GLU143, GLU151, GLU158, GLU195 and basic monomers of chain A: ARG111, ARG133, ARG137, ARG151, ARG173, HSP115, HSP122, HSP159, LYS5, LYS19, LYS56, LYS67, LYS78, LYS93, LYS100, LYS155, LYS166, LYS199. Lesser salt bridge interactions were not recorded.

In addition to measuring all salt bridge pairs (and hydrogen bond pairs), they were plotted over time (Figure 4A). A representative plot shows the interaction pairs that form with the acidic residue, Aspartic acid 8, during the 3ns simulation. As example, Asp8 from monomer A interacts with basic residues in chain B at Arginine111 (at t=1ns), Lysine67 (at t=1.5ns), Lysine56 (at t=1.82ns), and Lysine166 (at t=3ns). The plot in Figure 4A shows the range of values from 2.5 to 4.2Å in distance between possible salt bridge pairs. Figure 4B shows a particular example: in panel 1, Aspartic acid 173 is in hydrogen bond formation with polar Gln203 at a distance of 3.18 Å (at t=230ps). In panel 2, over the next 15ps, Asp173 partially breaks its hydrogen bond with Gln203 and forms a partial hydrogen bond to Lysine199. In panel 3, during the next 15ps, Asp173 only maintains a bond to Lys199 at a distance of 2.68Å (t=260ps). In panel 4, by t=275ps, Asp173 is losing its bond with Lys199 and moving to the next residue (Gln 195). In this way, the 'salt walking' and 'h-bond walking' progress along the X-Y plane in a circular path from one set of contact pairs to the next. We found similar salt walking properties among the other models. In addition, there are also helical openings that expose the side chains during rotation, which are discussed below.

III.6. Detailed Analysis of the Conformations

Figure 5A shows the energies for several simulations plotted for their interaction energies between the two protein monomers of lipid-bound ApoA-I discoidal complex. The total energy and interaction energy are composites of the electrostatic and VdW energies, since those are the two dominant energy contributors. The VdW contribution was nominal and is indicated to be only 20% of the total energy. The low peaks indicate the stable conformations, which are a result of strong salt bridge interaction. Indicated in Supplemental Figure S1, the Paris and Milan mutations are a two of the lower peaks. Examining the energetics on a per residue basis yields, the Paris (R151C registration) occurring at time = 1.13ns with an E = -3.73kcal/mol, and the Milano (R173C) occurred at time = 0.488ns and E = -4.22kcal/mol.

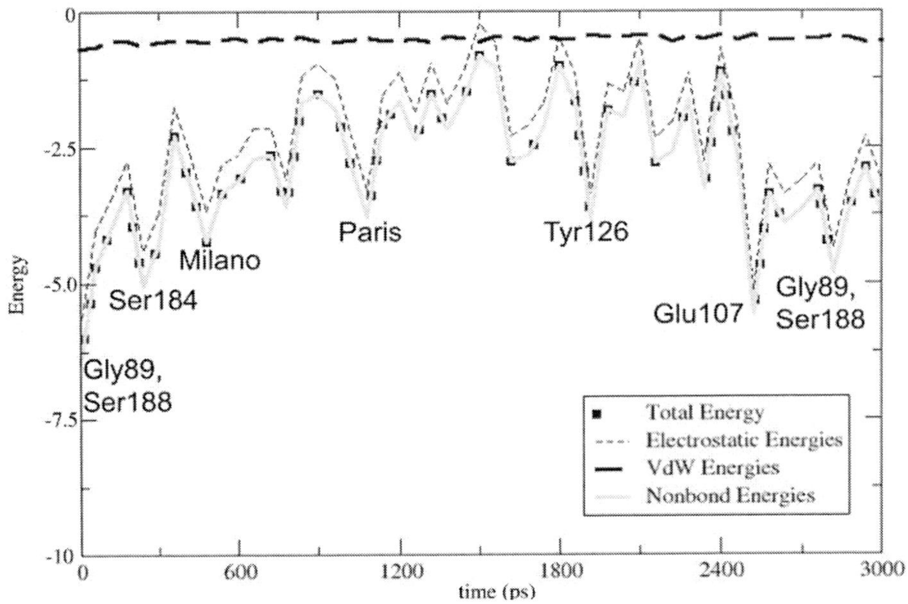

Figure 6. Energies of stable conformers. The interaction energies for the two protein monomers of the ampipathic α-helical ApoA-I calculated over 3ns simulation time. The Paris (R173C) and Milano (R151C) mutation locations occur at time = 490 ps and 1.13 ns, respectively. Tyr126 exhibits similar energetic properties at time = 1.92 ns. Improved energetic conformations were observed at Ser184 (t=150ps), Glu107 (t=2.52ns), and Gly89/Ser188 (t=0 and 2.82ns). The energies spread over all 203 residues, accounts for around 2.46 to 4 kcal/mol, likely sufficient to overcome thermal barriers. The side chains do not have identical orientation during rotation, leading side chain conformations to vary.

However, these are not the lowest energetic conformations revealed from the simulation. Three additional conformations were observed to have lower energies. Using registration nomenclature, Serine184 is aligned in both monomer A and B at t=0.1-0.15ns, where the energy is -4.92 kcal/mol. Tyr has an energy of -3.82 kcal/mol at t=1.92ns. Glu107 has an energy of -5.67 kcal/mol at t=2.52ns. Interestingly, Gly89-Gly89 and Ser188-Ser188 self aligns twice during the simulation: first at t=0ns with the E = -6.26 kcal/mol, and second at t=2.82ns with E = -4.87 kcal/mol. We do not suggest Ser184, Gly89, Ser188, or Glu107 are most favorable residues for Cys mutations to occur, but rather these registrations seem to have an optimal salt bridge score (see Discussion). For the sake of experimental clarity, we did examine a Glu107Cys mutant for any energetic differences from the native sequence. There is some indication that the cysteine mutant is more favorable. The results for this are shown in Figure 5A and Figure 5B and discussed above.

Concluding Remarks on the Findings from MdMD Biasing Methods for Probing ApoA-I Structural Arrangement during Dynamic Remodeling Events

Literature data on the two alpha-helical monomers was based on salt bridge scoring for various alignments [14]; demonstrating preferred specific registrations, e.g. the L5/5, Milano mutant, or Paris mutant [15]. The data form those studies salt bridge scoring data supported a double belt model and X-ray crystal structure observed [9, 13]. Current information confirms the important Paris and Milano mutants form a disulfide bridge at residues 151 and 173, respectively [16]. The Paris and Milano mutants indicate a change must be available to find proper registration. One proposed change is a rotationally circular movement of the protein monomers developed at the unilamellar bilayer. The mutants that possess cysteine in place of the arginine residue may lock the lipoprotein into a fixed conformation with chemical modifications.

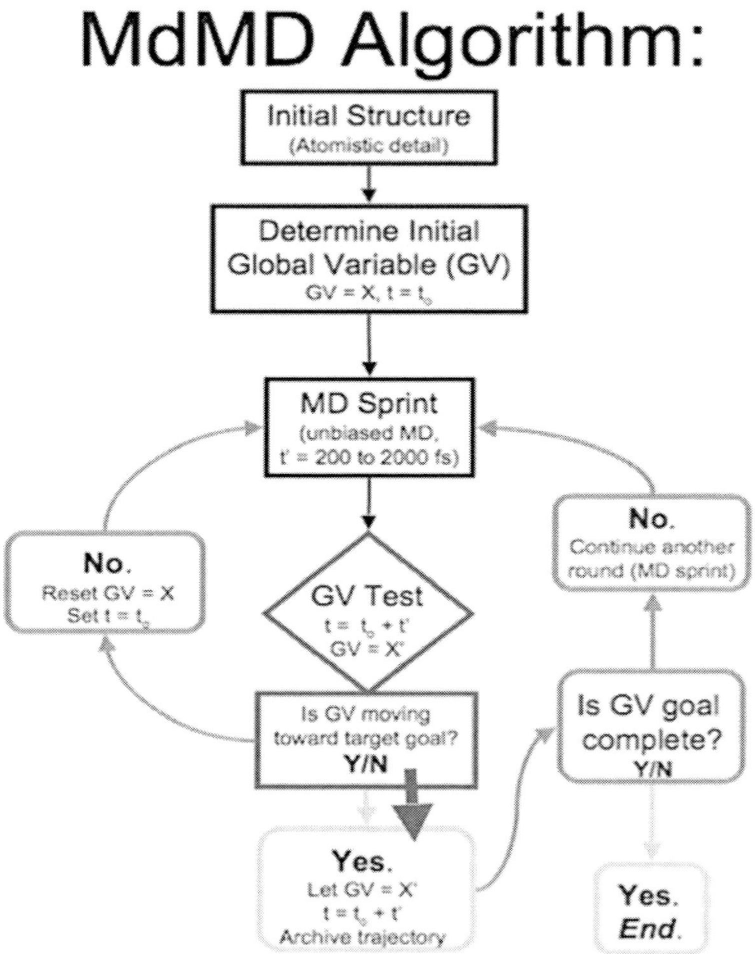

Figure 7. Flowchart for Maxwell's demon molecular dynamics. A schematic representation for the MdMD biasing algorithm.

Here, we described new work recently publishd that supports the existing double-belt model [16]. The salt bridge patterns found in the *monomer-to-monomer* ('salt walking') data suggest a method for conformational switching during discoidal formation of apolipoprotein A-I HDL. The data resulting from that new study finds a geometric sliding relationship along the edge of the POPC lipid bilayer that allows for the protein to accommodate for the influx of additional POPC lipids [16]. This lateral mode of sliding would allow for the registration of the two ampipathic α-helix protein chains to alter significantly allowing Milano and Paris mutants to search for the registration that allows the cysteine mutants to form a disulfide bond [16]. Two remarkable features of this simulation and generated models are: the well-maintained inter-helical geometry and favorable energetic scoring indicating alternate conformations. The wild-type does not maintain the lowest salt bridge score throughout the simulation [16]. The wild type conformation occurs at t=0ns and t=2.82ns. By 2.82ns, the score is no more favorable than that of Paris or Milano mutant registration. The lowest score is for Glu107-Glu107 registration. It is well known that the Paris and Milano mutations are exactly 22 residues apart in the sequence. Interestingly, Glu107 is positioned exactly two 22-mers from the Paris Mutant (R151) and three 22-mers from the Milano mutant (R173). The abundance of salt bridges observed for the Milano mutant and Paris mutant conformations are particularly favorable [14, 20, 24], and this is one reason for the low energy observed by the stabilizing presence of the abundance of salt bridges. Likewise, they find Glu107 has an abundance of salt bridges that lowers the energy significantly (Figure 5). Also, the wild type shown in previous salt bridge scoring metrics is considered very favorable [15]. But, after 3 nanoseconds of simulation and over a 400° rotation of the two protein monomers, there is a suggestion that the wild type is not more favorable than the Paris or Milan mutants (Figure 5). Without an uphill energetic cost, it is plausible that the conformational switch from wild type to the Paris or Milano mutation is not insurmountable. Likewise, Glu107 seems to be energetically favorable by comparison [16].

Figure 1C and Supplemental Movie S3 show the opening between monomers of the alpha-helices that form the discoidal complex of lipid-bound apo A-I. In these instances, the rotational motion contributes to release of the salt bridges, temporary interaction with the solvent, and lateral motion allowing new salt bridges to form. The slower rotating systems have more solvent exposure time, whereas the quickly rotating idealized system moved too quick for out-of-plane deformation and solvent disruptions. It appears that solvent disruptions may play a key role in allowing the two monomers to release from interaction and find new pairings [16]. Figure 5A scoring of low energy conformations may be useful for determining experimental tests of mutants. Similarities between the Milano and Paris mutant ApoA-I salt bridge scoring, the 22-mer periodicity, and energetic scoring shown in Fig. 6 predicts that Glu107 could be used to generate a viable mutant. The substitution of a cysteine residue for glutamic acid 107 should generate a mutant with similar structural and functional properties to the Paris and Milano ApoA-I mutants. Figure 5B does not demonstrate the same energy profile for the mutant although the native sequence is similar. The slower rate or rotation and longer sampling time allowed other more opportunistic interactions to dominate side chain interactions. And, there were much more substantial inter-helical disruptions allowing solvent to participate during rotation than in the native sequence case (Supplemental Movie S3). And, there are indications from the mutant simulation that reaffirms the strength of the Milano mutant. However, at the MdMD run time of 3 ns (300 ns MD sampling time), there seems to be confirmation of the Glu107Cys mutant. Interest in testing the Glu107Cys mutant may be noteworthy an effort considering the indication of it's strong interaction. Also noteworthy is the recent work of Segrest and co-workers coarse-grained approach on formation of spherical particles starting from discoidal models [48]. One area that could be additionally explored is the failure for the spherical-type particles to form in the case of the disulfide bridge with the Paris and Milano mutants, and with the proposed mutants here.

References

[1] Segrest, J.P., Jackson, R.L., Morrisett, J.D., Gotto Jr., A.M. A molecular theory of lipid—protein interactions in the plasma lipoproteins. *FEBS Lett.* 1974, 38, 247-53.

[2] Atkinson, D., Davis, M.A., Leslie, R.B. The structure of a high density lipoprotein (HDL3) from porcine plasma. *Proc. Natl. Acad. Sci. USA*. 1974, 186, 165-80.

[3] Brouillette, C.G., Anantharamaiah, G.M. Structural models of human apolipoprotein A-I. *Biochim. Biophys. Acta*. 1995, 1256, 103-29.

[4] Aakerloef, E., Joernvall, H., Slotte, H., Pousette, A. Identification of apolipoprotein-A1 and immunoglobulin as components of a serum complex that mediates activation of human sperm motility. *Biochemistry*. 1991, 30, 8986-90.

[5] Zhou, W., Ross, M.M., Tessitore, A., Ornstein, D., Vanmeter, A., Liotta, L.A., et al. An initial characterization of the serum phosphoproteome. *Proteome Res*. 2009, 8, 5523-31.

[6] Castelli, W.P.R., Garrison, P.W.F., Wilson, R.D., Abbott, S.K., Kannel, W.B. Incidence of coronary heart disease and lipoprotein cholesterol levels. *Journal Of the American Medical Association.* 1986, 256, 2835-8.

[7] Miller, G.J., Miller, N.E. Plasma-high-density-lipoprotein concentration and development of ischaemic heart disease. *Lancet*. 1975, i.

[8] Miller, N.E., Thelle, D.S., Förde, O.H., Mjös, O.D. The Tromso Heart Study: high-density lipoprotein and coronary heart disease: a prospective case-control study. *Lancet*. 1977, i.

[9] Wlodawer, A., Segrest, J.P., Chung, B.H., Chiovetti jr., R., Weinstein, J.N. High-density lipoprotein recombinants: evidence for a bicycle tire micelle structure obtained by neutron scattering and electron microscopy. *FEBS Lett*. 1979, 104, 231-5.

[10] Atkinson, D., Small, D.M., Shipley, G.G. X-ray and neutron scattering studies of plasma lipoproteins. *Ann. N.Y. Acad. Sci*. 1980, 348, 284-98.

[11] Jonas, A., Wald, J.H., Toohill, K.L., Krul, E.S., Kezdy, K.E. Apolipoprotein A-I structure and lipid properties in homogeneous, reconstituted spherical and discoidal high density lipoproteins. *Journal of Biological Chemistry*. 1990, 265, 22123-9.

[12] Monti, D.M., Guglielmi, F., Monti, M., Cozzolino, F., Torrassa, S., Relini, A., et al. Effects of a lipid environment on the fibrillogenic pathway of the N-terminal polypeptide of human apolipoprotein A-I, responsible for in vivo amyloid fibril formation. *European Biophysics Journal*. 2009, 39, 1289-99.

[13] Borhani, D.W., Rogers, D.P., Engler, J.A., Brouillette, C.G. Crystal structure of truncated human apolipoprotein A-I suggests a lipid-bound conformation. *Proc. Natl. Acad. Sci. USA*. 1997, 94, 12285-90.

[14] Segrest, J.P., Jones, M.K., Klon, A.E., Sheldahl, C.J., Hellinger, M., De Loof, H., et al. A Detailed Molecular Belt Model for Apolipoprotein A-I in Discoidal High Density Lipoprotein. *Journal of Biological Chemistry*. 1999, 274, 31755-8.

[15] Klon, A.E., Jones, M.K., Segrest, J.P., HArvey, S.C. Molecular Belt Models for the Apolipoprotein A-I Paris and Milano Mutations. *Biophysical Journal*. 2000, 79, 1679-85.

[16] Caulfield T. Inter-ring rotation of apolipoprotein A-I protein monomers for the double-belt model using biased molecular dynamics. *J. Molec. Graph. Modelling*. 2011, 29:1006-1014. PMID: 21570882.

[17] Heller, H., Schaefer, M., Schulten, K. Molecular dynamics simulation of a bilayer of 200 lipids in the gel and in the liquid-crystal phases. *Journal of Chemical Physics*. 1993, 97, 8843-360.

[18] Palgunachari, M.N., Mishra, V.K., Lund-Katz, S., Phillips, M.C., Adeyeye, S.O., Alluri, S., et al. Only the Two End Helixes of Eight Tandem Amphipathic Helical Domains of Human ApoA-I Have Significant Lipid Affinity : Implications for HDL Assembly. *Arteriosclerosis, Thrombosis, and Vascular Biology*. 1996, 16, 328-38.

[19] Mishra, V.K., Palgunachari, M.N. Interaction of Model Class A1, Class A2, and Class Y Amphipathic Helical Peptides with Membranes. *Biochemistry*. 1996, 35, 11210-20.

[20] Jones, M.K., Anantharamaiah, G.M., Segrest, J.P. Computer programs to identify and classify amphipathic alpha helical domains. *Journal of Lipid Research*. 1992, 287-96.

[21] Segrest, J.P., De Loof, H., Dohlman, J.G., Brouillette, C.G., Anantharamaiah, G.M. Amphipathic helix motif: Classes and properties. *Proteins*. 1990, 8, 103-17.

[22] Weisgraber, K.H., Rall, J., S.C., Bersot, T.P., Mahley, R.W., Franceschini, G., Sirtori, C.R. Apolipoprotein A-I(Milano). *Journal of Biological Chemistry*. 1983, 258, 2508-13.

[23] Bruckert, E.A., Funke, E.H., Beucler, I., Wiebusch, H., Turpin, G., Assmann, G. The replacement of arginine by cysteine at residue 151 in apolipoprotein A-I Milano produces a phenotype similar to that of apolipoprotein A-I. *Arteriosclerosis, Thrombosis, and Vascular Biology*. 1997, 128, 121-8.

[24] Rocco, A.G., Mollica, L., Gianazza, E., Calabresi, L., Franceschini, G., Sirtori, C.R., et al. Model Structure for the Heterodimer apoA-IMilano–apoA-II Supports Its Peculiar Susceptibility to Proteolysis. *Biophys. J.* 2006, 91, 3043-9.

[25] Calabresi, L.G., Franceschi, A., Burkybile, A., Jonas, A. Activation of lecithin cholesterol acyltransferase by a disulfide-linked apolipoprotein A-I dimer. *Biochem. Biophys. Res. Commun.* 1997, 232, 345-9.

[26] Franceschini, G., Calabresi, L.G., Chiesa, G., Parolini, C., Sirtori, C.R., Canavesi, M., et al. Increased cholesterol efflux potential of sera from ApoA-I(Milano) carriers and transgenic mice. *Journal of Clinical Investigation*. 1999, 66, 892-900.

[27] Daum, U., Lanager, C., Duverger, N., Emmanuel, F., Benoit, P., Denefle, P., et al. Apolipoprotein A-I(R151C)Paris is defective in activation of lecithin: cholesterol acyltransferase but not in initial lipid binding, formation of reconstituted lipoproteins, or promotion of cholesterol efflux. *Journal of Molecular Medicine*. 1999, 77.

[28] Pérusse, M., Pascot, A., Després, J.P., Couillard, C., Lamarche, B. A new method for HDL particle sizing by polyacrylamide gradient gel electrophoresis using whole plasma. *J. Lipid Res.* 2001, 42, 1331-4.

[29] Klon, A.E., Segrest, J.P., Harvey, S.C. Comparative models for human apolipoprotein a-I bound to lipid in discoidal high-density lipoprotein particles. *Biochemistry*. 2002, 41, 10895-905.

[30] Accelrys, I. Accelrys Inc., 9685 Scranton Road, San Diego, California 92121, USA. amaiti@accelrys.com. INSIGHT-II. 2000.

[31] Humphrey, W., Dalke, A., Schulten, K. VMD: visual molecular dynamics. *J. Mol. Graph.* 1996, 14, 33-8, 27-8.

[32] Krawetz, J.P., Shinozaki, A., Varadarajan, K., and Schulten, K. NAMD2: Greater scalability for parallel molecular dynamics. *Journal of Computational Physics*. 1999, 151, 283-312.

[33] Nelson, M., Humphrey, W., Gursoy, A., Dalke, A., Kalé, L., Skeel, R.D., et al. NAMD - A parallel object-oriented molecular dynamics program. *J. Supercomput. Appl.* 1996, 10, 251-68.

[34] Jones, M.K., Catte, A., Li, L., Segrest, J.P. Dynamics of lecithin:cholesterol acyltransferase activation by apolipoprotein A-I. *Biochemistry*. 2009, 48, 11196.

[35] Klon, A.E., Jones, M.K., Segrest, J.P., Harvey, S.C. Molecular Belt Models for the Apolipoprotein A-I Paris and Milano Mutations. *Biophys. J.* 2000, 79, 1679-85.

[36] Jones, M.K., Catte, A., Patterson, J.C., Gu, F., Chen, J., Li, L., et al. Thermal Stability of Apolipoprotein A-I in High-Density Lipoproteins by Molecular Dynamics. 96. 2009, 2, 354-71.

[37] Catte, A., Patterson, J.C., Jones, M.K., Jerome, W.G., Bashtovyy, D., Su, Z., et al. Novel Changes in Discoidal High Density Lipoprotein Morphology: A Molecular Dynamics Study. *Biophys. J.* 2006, 90, 4345-60.

[38] Jorgensen, W.L., Chandrasekhar, J., Madura, J.D., Impey, R.W., Klein, M.L. Comparison of simple potential functions for simulating liquid water. *Journal of Chemical Physics*. 1983, 79, 926-35.

[39] Brooks, B.R., Olafson, R.E.B., States, D.J., Swaminathan, S., Karplus, M. CHARMM: A Program for Macromolecular Energy, Minimization, and Dynamics Calculations. *J. Comput. Chem.* 1983, 4, 187-217.

[40] Ryckaert, J., Ciccotti, G., Berendsen, H. SHAKE: Numerical Integration of the Cartesian Equations of Motion of a System with Constraints: Molecular Dynamics of n-Alkanes. *Journal of Computational Physics*. 1977, 23, 327-41.

[41] Darden., T., York, D., Pedersen, L. Paticle Mesh Ewald--an N.Log(N) method for Ewald sums in large systems. *Journal of Chemical Physics*. 1993, 98, 10089-92.

[42] Nosé, E. A unified formulation of the constant temperature molecular dynamics method. *Journal of Chemical Physics*. 1984, 81, 511-9.

[43] Hooover, W.G. Canonical dynamics: Equilibrium phase-space distributions. *Physical Review A*. 1985, 31, 1695-7.

[44] Berendsen, H.J.C., Postma, J., Van Gunsteren, W., Dinola, A., Haak, J. Molecular-Dynamics with Coupling to an External Bath. *Journal of Chemical Physics*. 1984, 81, 3684-90.

[45] Caulfield, T., Devkota, B., Rollins, G. Examinations of tRNA range of motion using simulations of cryo-EM microscopy and X-ray data. *Journal of Biophysics*. 2011, in press.

[46] Harvey, S.C., Gabb, H.A. Conformational transitions using molecular dynamics with minimum biasing. *Biopolymers*. 1993, 33, 1167-72.

[47] Gu, F., Jones, M.K., Chen, J., Patterson, J.C., Catte, A., Jerome, W.G., et al. Structures of Discoidal High Density Lipoproteins: A Combined Computational-Experimental Approach. *Journal of Biological Chemistry*. 2010, 285, 4652-65.

[48] Catte, A., Patterson, J.C., Bashtovyy, D., Jones, M.K., Gu, F., Li, L., et al. Structure of spheroidal HDL particles revealed by combined atomistic and coarse-grained simulation. *Biophys. J.* 2008, 94, 2306.

In: Apolipoproteins
Editors: A. D. Sidorov and M. Y. Nikitin
ISBN: 978-1-62257-484-1

Chapter III

Understanding the Role of Apolipoprotein E in Cardiovascular and Renal Diseases

***C. M. Balarini*[1], *I. B. S. Gomes*[2], *E. C. Vasquez*[1,4], *S. S. Meyrelles*[1,3] *and A. L. Gava*[1,3]**

[1]Physiological Sciences Graduate Program, Federal University of Espirito Santo, Vitória, ES, Brazil

[2]Pharmaceutical Sciences Department, Federal University of Espirito Santo, Vitória, ES, Brazil

[3]Biotechnology Graduate Program, Federal University of Espirito Santo, Vitória, ES, Brazil

[4]Emescam Healthy Sciences School, Vitória, ES, Brazil

Abstract

It is well established that apolipoproteins play a crucial role in serum lipids transport and metabolism. Particularly, the apolipoprotein E (apoE) is mainly involved in the transport of very-low density lipoproteins and intermediary density lipoproteins by the liver, but new insights revealed a wide range of functions performed by apoE. This lipoprotein is related to the modulation of inflammatory process and regulates the expression of multiple genes in various diseases. Besides, apoE isoforms are involved in progression of cardiovascular and renal diseases. Here we present a review about the achievements in both experimental and clinical studies that contribute to understanding the role of apoE in both physiological and pathological situations. We focus in the participation of apoE as a key modulatory factor to the development of atherosclerosis, diabetes and kidney diseases and the contributions of available animal models to clarify the mechanisms involved in these pathologies in humans.

Introduction

Lipids are important molecules to the normal functioning of the body, since these substances can act as energy store, cell membrane components, hormones, intracellular messengers, enzymatic co-factors, electron transporters and others. Biochemically, lipids are characterized by their insolubility in water. In the plasma these molecules are transported in a soluble complex, called lipoprotein, containing a unique protein component, the apolipoprotein.

There are about 12 different types of apolipoproteins, grouped in five main types (A, B, C, D and E) (Eichner et al., 2002), involved in the transportation and binding of the several lipoproteins in specific tissues. Particularly, the apolipoprotein E (apoE), which was first described in 1973 (Shore and Shore, 1973), mediates the uptake of chylomicrons (CM) and very-low density lipoprotein (VLDL) and their remnants, such as the intermediary density lipoprotein (IDL), by the liver through interaction with members of the low-density lipoprotein (LDL) receptor family (Kolovou et al., 2008; Hauser et al., 2011).

The main function of lipoproteins is to transport triglycerides and cholesterol from their exogenous (intestine) and endogenous (liver) sources to the tissues where they will be used to produce energy or to be stored. Lipids obtained from diet are transported in the blood as CM, which are considered triglycerides (TG)-rich particles and present apoB-48 as their major apolipoprotein. On the other hand, TG produced by the liver reaches the blood as VLDL, an apoB-100 containing particle. Both CM and VLDL also contain apoE and acquire apoC in the serum. The release of TG to the cells is mediated by the action of lipoprotein lipase (stimulated by apoC) in vascular endothelium, generating remnant CM and IDL, respectively. These remnant particles are internalized in the liver through the LDL receptor binding to apoE (Dominiczak and Caslake, 2011).

TG-rich particles (CM and VLDL) can also transfer some TG to the high-density lipoprotein (HDL), in exchange for cholesteryl esters, in a process mediated by the enzyme cholesteryl ester transfer protein (CETP) (Bachorik et al., 2008). In the liver microvasculature, the hepatic TG lipase transforms the excess of VLDL and IDL in LDL, which contains apoB-100 as the main apolipoprotein and controls LDL internalization by binding to the LDL receptor. Once there are some relevant structural differences between this apoB-100 and apoB-48, the latter is not capable of binding to LDL receptor (Hui et al., 1984).

The binding of apoB-100 to LDL receptor initiates the process of uptake and degradation of this particle, leading to the use of the cholesterol content in the regulation of intracellular cholesterol metabolism (Mahley, 1988). Briefly, once lipoprotein binds to the LDL receptor in cell surface and the complex is uptaken, the release of this exogenous cholesterol into intracellular space decreases the syntesis of endogenous cholesterol by inhibition of 3-hydroxy-3-methyl-glutaryl-CoA reductase (HMG-CoA reductase) and the expression of LDL receptor in the cell surface, reducing the influx of more LDL. These discoveries concerning the regulation of cholesterol metabolism gave Michael S. Brown and Joseph L. Goldstein the Nobel Prize in Physiology or Medicine in 1985.

The cell membrane derived cholesterol is captured by HDL and esterified by lecithin-cholesterol acyltransferase (LCAT). This esterified cholesterol can be transferred to VLDL or LDL under the action of CETP or transported into the liver by HDL. It is important to notice that both VLDL and IDL present apoE in the surface of the molecule, which mediates the

LDL receptor-mediated clearance of these particles. Moreover, apoE is also involved in reverse cholesterol transport mediated by HDL and this dual role of this apolipoprotein is crucial for clearing the plasma from cholesterol excess (Anoop et al., 2010).

ApoE is a 34 kDa glycoprotein synthesized by the liver, brain, kidney and other tissues and it is composed by 299 aminoacids in humans (Elshourbagy et al., 1985; Jawien et al., 2004; Hauser et al., 2011). ApoE is the major ligand for two types of receptors: the LDL receptor (also called B/E receptor), found in liver and other tissues and apoE-specific receptor, present in the liver. The carboxi terminal region of the protein mediates the binding of apoE to the lipoprotein surface and the amino terminal is responsible for binding it to the LDL receptor (Greenow et al., 2005).

ApoE is not only involved in the regulation of cholesterol metabolism. Recent studies demonstrate that apoE carries out additional functions, such as stimulation of cholesterol efflux from macrophages, prevention of platelet aggregation, inhibition of T-lymphocytes, endothelial cells and smooth muscular cells proliferation, inhibition of lipid oxidation, stimulation of synapse formation, nerve regeneration and modulation of inflammatory and imune responses (Hauser et al., 2011; Greenow et al., 2005; Zhang et al., 2011).

In this review we focus in the participation of apoE as a key modulator factor to the development of atherosclerosis, diabetes and kidney diseases and the contributions of available animal models to the understanding of the mechanisms involved in these pathologies in humans.

Apolipoprotein E and Atherosclerosis

Cardiovascular diseases have become a public health problem worldwide. According to the World Health Organization (WHO), 30% of the deaths in 2008 occurred due to diverse forms of cardiovascular events. Most of the cardiovascular deaths can be attributed to atherosclerosis and its complications. In westernized societies, atherosclerosis is the underlying cause of about 50% of all deaths (Lusis, 2000).

Atherosclerosis can be defined as a progressive inflammatory disease of the arterial wall, characterized by the accumulation of lipids, inflammatory cells and fibrous elements in the large arteries, which progresses to thrombosis as a final complication (Libby, 2002; Libby et al., 2010; Libby et al., 2011). High serum cholesterol, in particular in LDL form, is the most important risk factor for plaque deposition (Ross, 1999).

Atherogenesis process initiates with an altered permeability of the arterial wall (Gerrity, 1981), leading to extracellular deposition of lipids (Simionescu et al., 1986). This process is accompanied by endothelial dysfunction (Kharbanda and MacAllister, 2005; Meyrelles et al., 2011), possibly caused by elevated and modified LDL, excess of free radicals, genetic alterations, elevated plasma homocysteine concentrations, infectious microorganisms and combinations of these and other factors (Ross, 1999). Endothelial dysfunction increment the expression of mediators involved in recruitment of leucocytes (monocytes and T cells) and their adhesion and migration through endothelial surface. Once in subendothelial space, monocytes mature into macrophages, which express scavenger receptors that mediate the phagocytosis of modified lipoprotein particles, leading to the transformation of macrophages into foam cells (Gerrity, 1981; Libby et al., 2010) and generating fatty streaks in arterial wall.

Additionally, lipoproteins accumulated in the intima layer suffer a variety of modifications that can alter their structure and favor the internalization by non-scavenger receptor-mediated pathways (Moore et al., 2005).

Atheroma formation also involves the recruitment and proliferation of smooth muscle cells (SMC) into the tunica intima. In response to platelet-derived growth factor released by activated macrophages and endothelial cells, SMC migrate from the tunica media to the tunica intima, where they proliferate under the stimuli of various growth factors (Packard and Libby, 2008). SMC produce extracellular matrix, such as collagen and elastin, forming a fibrous cap that overlies a necrotic and lipid-rich core, which often compromises the vascular lumen (Tabas, 2010). The fact that the progression of atherosclerotic lesions is similar in different experimental models with different genotypes reinforces the idea that the sequence of events that allow the transformation of fatty streaks into advanced plaques is similar, regardless the cause of hyperlipidemia (Reddick et al., 1994).

The major determinants of the inter-individual variation in susceptibility to development of atherosclerosis includes genetic polymorphism of apolipoproteins, since these molecules play a pivotal role in modulating lipoprotein plasma concentrations and its metabolic pathways (Davignon et al., 1988). ApoE gene polymorphism contributes more to normal cholesterol variability than any other gene identified involved in cholesterol metabolism (Sing and Davignon, 1985).

The gene encoding apoE is located in chromosome 19 and the polymorphic protein has three common isoforms (E2, E3 e E4) and more than 20 rare variants (Rall et al., 1992). E2, E3 and E4 are encoded respectively by the alleles ε2, ε3 and ε4, generating six different possible phenotypes: E2/2, E2/3, E2/4, E3/3, E3/4 and E4/4 (Greenow et al., 2005). The E3 variant is the most frequent (Eichner et al., 2002). These isoforms differs from each other in amino acid positions 112 and 158. E2 isoform presents cysteine at both positions, while E3 contains cysteine at 112 and arginine at 158 and E4 has arginine at both sites (Weisgraber et al., 1981). Although the apoE isoforms differ from each other by only two amino acid substitutions, these changes have profound effects on structural and functional levels (Greenow et al., 2005), such as the affinity for binding to the LDL receptor and the lipoprotein particles (Davignon et al., 1988). While considering experimental models, it is important to mention that mouse apoE contains arginine in a position equivalent to 112 in human apoE, but instead of arginine in the position 61, there is a threonine. This confers to the mouse apoE a functionality equivalent to the human apoE3 (Huang, 2010).

Apolipoprotein ε2 allele is associated with higher concentrations of apoE and ε4 with lower concentrations (Siest et al., 1995). Carriers of ε2 allele are less efficient at making and transferring VLDL and CM from the blood to the liver because of its binding properties, while carriers of the ε3 and ε4 alleles are more efficient in these processes (Eichner et al., 2002). It is interesting to notice that affinity of apoE2 isoform to LDL receptor is less than 2% of the affinity of apoE3 and apoE4 (Innerarity et al., 1984). This is due to the absence of arginine amino acid at position 158, which is occupied by cysteine in E2 isoform (Lalazar et al., 1988), resulting in differences in regulating LDL receptors and contributing to differences in total and LDL cholesterol levels (Eichner et al., 2002). Because of the lower affinity of apoE2 to LDL receptor, a reduction in cellular cholesterol influx occurs, leading to LDL accumulation in the serum and to an up regulation of LDL receptor. The apoE4 is preferentially present in TG-rich particles and accelerates its uptake, leading to down regulation of hepatic LDL receptor, thereby causing increased levels of LDL (Mahley and

Rall, 2000). Studies have shown that populations with higher cholesterol levels and increased coronary heart disease mortality rates have an augmented frequency of apoE4, suggesting that patients who carry this genotype are more prone to develop cardiovascular complications (Eichner et al., 2002).

ApoE is also involved in regulation of smooth muscle cells proliferation and migration into the intima, due to its capacity of binding to heparin and heparin-like glycosoaminoglycans present in the matrix of arterial walls (Anoop et al., 2010). Moreover, it stimulates the cholesterol efflux from macrophages, prevents platelet aggregation and inhibits proliferation of T-lymphocytes and endothelial cells (Greenow et al., 2005).

Considering the important role played by apoE in lipid metabolism and atheroma formation, in 1992 two different research groups created the apoE knockout mouse (apoE$^{-/-}$) using homologous recombination to inactivate apoE gene in embryonic stem cells (Plump et al., 1992; Piedrahita et al, 1992). It is important to notice that the lack of apoE is compatible with normal development and that the homozygous animals have been born at the expected frequency (Piedrahita et al., 1992), which allows this model to be bred in research laboratories.

Since apoE serves as the ligand that mediates the uptake of CM and VDLD and their remnants through LDL receptor, the lack of this protein impairs the clearing of lipoproteins (Kolovou et al., 2008). ApoE$^{-/-}$ mice present higher levels of plasma cholesterol when compared to wild-type animals. The lipid profile in mice differs from that in humans, who carry most of the serum cholesterol in LDL particles. Normally, mice do not express CETP and thus carry most of their plasma cholesterol in HDL particles (Li et al., 2011a). However apoE$^{-/-}$ mice lipid profile resembles that found in humans, once they present a shift in plasma lipoprotein from HDL to cholesterol-rich remnants of CM and VLDL (Jawien et al., 2004).

The analysis of atherogenic process in apoE$^{-/-}$ reveals that the sequential events involved in lesion formation in this model are similar to those found in well-established larger animal models of atherosclerosis and in humans (Nakashima et al., 1994). Atherosclerotic lesions in this model locates, preferentially in the aortic root, aortic arch, common carotid, superior mesenteric artery, renal and pulmonary arteries and the process of atherogenesis and severity of lesions can be accelerated by a hyperlipidemic Western-type diet (Vasquez et al., 2012). In young animals, early lesions consist of foam cells, while in older animals, fibrous-cap lesions are observed, covered by smooth muscle cells (Reddick et al., 1994). For a long time it was believed that murine models of atherosclerosis did not present plaque rupture, which is fairly common in humans and, in fact, is the most concern event involving atherosclerosis. However, it has been shown that in older apoE$^{-/-}$ mice, brachiocephalic arterial plaques demonstrate features likely to be the murine parallel of vulnerable human plaques, including the presence of an acellular necrotic core, erosion of the necrotic mass through the lumen and intraplaque hemorrhage (Rosenfeld et al, 2000; Meir and Leitersdorf, 2004). Taken together, these data demonstrate that apoE$^{-/-}$ mice consist in an excellent model for studying atherogenesis, the relationship between genetic and environmental determinants of atherosclerosis and possible novel pharmacological and non-pharmacological interventions to reduce plaque deposition (Plump et al., 1992; Meir and Leitersdorf, 2004).

In addition to classical pathways involved in the atheroma formation, other mechanisms can contribute to plaque development in apoE-knockout mouse. It has already been reported that VLDL and IDL from apoE$^{-/-}$ mouse produce a significant cholesteryl ester accumulation in macrophages, leading to formation of foam cells through a specific and apoE-independent pathway (Zhang et al., 1999). Besides, it is well recognized that there is a positive correlation between plasma cholesterol and glycosphingolipids concentrations in humans. In apoE$^{-/-}$, there is an increase in serum concentrations of glycosphingolipids and accumulation of them in atherosclerosis-prone regions of the aorta (Kolovou et al., 2008). Local apoE production is also important to prevent atherosclerosis. ApoE expression through gene transfer into macrophages or into the blood vessel wall diminishes atherosclerosis through mechanisms independent of cholesterol-lowering effects (Shimano et al., 1995). Although these new mechanisms by which the lack of apoE contributes to atherosclerosis are not well defined, the role of apoE in maintaining the normal vascular homeostasis is an unquestionable fact.

Apolipoprotein E and Diabetes

Nowadays diabetes represents one of the most important healthcare challenge worldwide. The 21st century has the most diabetogenic environment in human history. In 2007, there were 246 million people with diabetes in the world, but by 2025, that number is forecast to reach 380 million. People with impaired glucose tolerance, a "prediabetic state", numbered 308 million in 2007 and will increase to 418 million by 2025. This increase in the prevalence of diabetes will be greater in the developing countries (Atkins et al., 2010).

The interaction between diabetes and cardiovascular diseases is the focus of many investigations. Epidemiological data have demonstrated the correlation between coronary heart disease and diabetes mellitus, since individuals with diabetes have 2-to-4-fold higher risk of developing micro and macrovascular complications and a 10-to-15-fold increased risk of a lower extremity amputation than non-diabetic individuals (D'Souza et al., 2009; Goraya et al., 2002). Additionally, diabetic patients frequently show accelerated atherosclerosis, undergo acute coronary syndromes, myocardial ischemia with peripheral artery disease and stroke (Peter et al., 2008). Therefore, cardiovascular diseases are the major cause of morbidity and mortality among diabetic patients (Haffer et al., 1998).

Diabetic patients often have abnormalities of lipid metabolism. Increases in VLDL triglycerides; decreases in HDL; the accumulation of smaller, more dense LDL; slower clearance of postprandial chylomicrons; and a decrease in LDL receptor (LDLR) expression are all noted phenotypes associated with both type 1 and type 2 diabetes (Goldberg, 2001). Recent research indicates that dyslipidemia frequently precedes type 2 diabetes mellitus for years, suggesting that changes in lipoprotein profile may initiate the pathological process leading to diabetes (Li et al., 2011b). It is interesting to notice that all of these components of diabetic dyslipidemia are areas of normal lipid metabolism in which apoE has previously been shown to play a direct role.

These disturbances in lipid metabolism are one of the major factors contributing to vascular diseases, such as atherosclerosis. Diabetic patients show reduced turnover of their LDL particles with a decreased catabolism, leading to rises in LDL plasma resident time, which seems to promote the deposition of cholesterol in the arterial wall. This impaired LDL catabolism in type 2 diabetes may occur as consequence of the reduction in the number of LDL B/E receptors (Vergès, 2009). For a better understanding of the mechanisms linking diabetes and atherogenesis, animal models has been used. An ideal animal model should have hyperglycemia associated with a lipid profile which promotes atherogenesis within an experimentally feasible amount of time (Kako et al., 2002).

The apoE-deficient (apoE$^{-/-}$) mouse is one of the most widely used experimental model of atherosclerosis. Treatment with streptozocin (STZ), a pancreatic β-cell toxin, significantly impairs the animal's ability to produce insulin and accelerates atherosclerosis, leading to a model of diabetic atherosclerosis (Calkin et al., 2006).

This model was first described by Park et al. (1998) in which the authors showed glycemia above 350mg/dL and a 5.3-fold increase in mean lesion area at the level of the aortic sinus and an two-fold increase in cholesterol plasma levels in diabetic apoE$^{-/-}$ mice compared with control mice 6 weeks after streptozocin treatment. Long-term studies described the effects of 20 weeks of diabetes in apoE$^{-/-}$ mice and the results showed a four-to-five-fold increase in total plaque area across the whole aorta (arch, thoracic and abdominal segments). Moreover, these lesions had an asymmetrically thickened intima composed of a fibrous cap with smooth muscle cells, foamy macrophages, and a lipid-rich necrotic core with cholesterol clefts within the extracellular matrix (Calkin et al., 2008; Candido et al., 2004; Candido et al., 2002).

Other mouse models of diabetic atherosclerosis include: streptozocin-induced diabetes in mice expressing human apolipoprotein B, with a heterozygous deletion of lipoprotein lipase and fed a Western diet; streptozocin-induced diabetes in low-density lipoprotein receptor (LDLR) knockout mice (LDLR$^{-/-}$) fed a Western diet; and LDLR$^{-/-}$ mice crossed with leptin-deficient mice. All of these models are associated with an extreme hyperlipidemia and thus, it has been difficult to assess if the increase in atherosclerosis is due to high lipid levels or diabetes *per se* (Calkin et al., 2006).

Insulin can activate several mechanisms considered proatherosclerotic through direct effects on vascular cells, including increased endothelial cell expression of endothelin-1 (Oliver et al., 1991; Cardillo et al., 1999) and plasminogen activator inhibitor-1 (Nordt et al., 1998; Grenett et al., 1998) and increased smooth muscle cell proliferation (Banskota et al., 1989). These insulin-induced effects have been postulated to mediate, at least in part, the acceleration of the atherosclerosis proccess during diabetes. However, a recent investigation demonstrated that hyperinsulinemia *per se* is not sufficient to speed up plaque deposition (Rask-Madsen et al., 2012). During the characterization of mice bred to create tissue-specific insulin receptor knockout, Rask-Madsen et al. (2010) created a mouse with whole-body knockout of a single allele of the insulin receptor combined with total knockout of the apoE gene. Metabolic studies showed that, compared with littermate controls, these mice had hyperinsulinemia primarily due to decreased insulin clearance, with no detectable impairment of insulin signaling and no change in glucose tolerance or whole-body insulin sensitivity measured by insulin tolerance tests, suggesting that they would be an attractive model for studying the effect of hyperinsulinemia on atherosclerosis development. The authors found no difference in atherosclerotic lesion size in hyperinsulinemic mice compared with controls. These data indicate that abnormally high insulin concentrations alone, without substantial impairment of vascular insulin signaling, and in the absence of significant changes in glucose or lipid metabolism, are not sufficient to accelerate atherosclerosis (Rask-Madsen et al., 2012). These results suggest that in the metabolic syndrome and type 2 diabetes, activation of potentially proatherosclerotic mechanisms in vascular cells by hyperinsulinemia has little effect on atherogenesis, whereas substantial insulin resistance in endothelial cells by itself can promote atherosclerosis development.

Epidemiological studies have suggested that in certain populations, apoE genotype may influence plasma glucose and insulin levels (Scuteri et al., 2005; Elosua et al., 2003), postprandial glucose response (Dart et al., 1997), the development of metabolic syndrome (Sima et al., 2007; Olivieri et al., 2007) and a myriad of diabetes complications (Freedman et al., 2007). Corroborating these data, Arbones-Mainar et al. (2008) demonstrated that mice expressing apoE4 are more susceptible to diet-induced glucose intolerance than those expressing apoE3 and that this propensity of apoE4 expressing mice to develop glucose intolerance likely contributes to the impaired lipid metabolism in the insulin-deficient state. ApoE4 carriers with diabetes have been shown to have increased carotid atherosclerosis (Elosua et al., 2004), and elderly apoE4 carriers with diabetes have an increased risk of CVD-associated death (Guang-da et al., 2004). Chaudhary et al. (2012) reported that people with ε4 allele presents a high risk of developing type 2 diabetes and coronary artery disease. Taken together, these data demonstrated that apoE4 genotype seems to be a risk factor to the development of both diabetes and atherosclerosis.

Apolipoprotein E and Kidney Diseases

It is well established that there is a strong association between cardiovascular and kidney diseases. Risk factors to the development of cardiovascular diseases, such as dyslipidemias, may also influence the progression of renal dysfunction. In fact, the prevalence of dyslipidemia in patients with chronic kidney disease (CKD) is much higher than in the general population whilst elevated cholesterol and triglyceride levels are associated with more rapid deterioration of kidney function (Schaeffner et al., 2003). On the other hand, the progressive decline of renal function in chronic kidney disease may also lead to dyslipidemia and contributes to the development of atherosclerosis (Maggori et al., 2003; Godin and Dahlman, 1993). Corroborating these data, atherosclerotic vascular lesions are more prevalent in CKD patients than in non-CKD patients. In this manner, dyslipidemia and atherosclerosis accelerate renal dysfunction, which in turn, promotes atherosclerosis. This vicious cycle is present even in moderate reductions of glomerular filtration rate (GFR), and therefore, patients with CKD are more likely to die of cardiovascular disease than to progress to end-stage renal disease (Weiner et al., 2006).

Considering that apoE plays an important role in normal lipid metabolism, several studies have hypothesized that disturbances in apoE production and/or functioning might take part in the pathogenesis of renal diseases. In renal tissue, apoE is mainly synthesized by mesangial cells and renal tubular epithelial cells under normal physiologic condition (Lin et al., 1986), and apoE receptors are present in endothelial, mesangial and visceral epithelial cells. Additionally, in the glomerulus these cells can take up the serum lipids by receptor independent-mechanism (Zhou et al., 2011a). Reverse transcriptase-polymerase chain reaction (RT-PCR) analysis showed that mesangial cells are the major source of apoE expression in the kidney and may serve as an autocrine regulator of such mesangial expansion. ApoE has anti-proliferative properties and inhibits mesangial proliferation induced by different stimuli including growth factors and lipids (Chen et al., 2001).

The deposition of lipids in glomeruli is involved in the formation and development of glomerulosclerosis. Some observations in experimental animals and microscopic examination of human renal biopsies support the concept that the lipid deposits might be involved in the pathological process of glomerular sclerosis (Grond et al.,1986; Boumendjel et al., 2010). The direct negative effects of lipid over-accumulation on the renal parenchymal cells is due to the formation of oxidized low-density lipoprotein (ox-LDL), which can induce mesangial cells and macrophages to release cytokines and growth factors (such as TGF-β1), leading to mesangial proliferation and extracellular matrix accumulation (Zhou et al., 2011a). Interestingly, the process of glomerulosclerosis, the hallmark of end stage renal disease (ESRD) in many kidney diseases, has common features with that of atherosclerosis (Diamond, 1991), such as endothelial dysfunction and unregulated cell proliferation. Glomerular inflammation, mesangial expansion, foam cell formation and endothelial activation have been found to occur in the kidney of apoE$^{-/-}$ mice (Bruneval et al., 2002; Wen et al., 2002; Bonomini et al., 2010; Vaziri et al,. 2010; Balarini et al., 2011). Therefore, apoE$^{-/-}$ mice provide an animal model suitable to study the effects of hyperlipidaemia on kidney disease.

Some authors have reported a protective role for apoE in preventing kidney diseases. In a recent study, Bonomini et al. (2010) evaluated the renal morphology in apoE$^{-/-}$ mice ranging from 6 to 20 weeks of age. The authors reported significant alterations in the kidneys of apoE$^{-/-}$ mice at all ages, such as interstitial fibrosis, glomerolusclerosis, tubular atrophy and Bowman's capsule dilation. It was also observed an increase of oxidative stress, increase of TNF-α and NF-kB and a decrease of antioxidant enzymes expression. Corroborating these data, Vaziri et al. (2010) demonstrated that apoE$^{-/-}$ mice present significant proteinuria, foam cell formation, occasional glomerular capillary thrombosis and significant glomerular and tubulo-interstitial macrophage and lymphocyte accumulation. On the other hand, studies also demonstrated a detrimental effect of apoE on renal function. On lipoprotein glomerulopathy, the most characteristic biochemical finding is the elevated serum concentration of apoE (Tsimihodimos and Elisaf, 2011). The light microscopic examination of renal specimens discloses dilated glomerular capillaries that have been occluded by a pale-stained amorphous material. Sudan or oil-red-O staining reveals lipid droplets in these intraluminal deposits, and in advanced cases segmental sclerosis and periglomerular and interstitial fibrosis are common (Tsimihodimos and Elisaf, 2011). In rat model of glomerulosclerosis, the animals present an elevated serum level of apoE and lipid accumulation in renal parenchyma cells in the glomerulus (Zhou et al., 2011b). The increased lipid deposition may also cause elevation of reactive oxygen species (ROS) generation (Dentelli et al., 2007), leading to glomerular injury. This impairment of renal parenchymal cells changes the permeability of glomerular basement membrane, increases mesangial proliferation and extracellular matrix accumulation (Zhou et al., 2011b).

Considering that the effects of apoE on the kidney are primarily attributed to its effects on lipid metabolism, the use of lipid lowering substances may provide an important pharmaceutical approach to treat dyslipidemia-induced kidney diseases. HMG-CoA (3-hydroxy-3-methyl-glutaryl-CoA reductase) inhibitors, generally called statins, are commonly used to lower serum total and low density lipoprotein cholesterol. They have proven efficacy in decreasing cardiovascular events in the general population (Pedersen et al., 2004). Even in the absence of cholesterol-lowering effects, statins may be beneficial in the treatment of atherosclerosis due to local anti-inflammatory and antioxidant actions. They may occur via the up-regulation of endothelial nitric oxide synthase with the increased bioavailability of nitric oxide, a decrease in cellular proliferation, an increase in apoptosis and/or an interference with local oxidative injury (Rikitake and Liao, 2005). Ivanovski et al. (2008) demonstrated that chronic kidney disease enhanced aortic plaque development in apoE$^{-/-}$ mice compared with controls and that simvastatin treatment did not reduce the atherosclerotic lesions in the aortic root or thoracic aorta in this experimental model, in line with its failure to decrease serum total cholesterol. Nevertheless, simvastatin therapy led to a significant decrease in intima calcium content, that is the calcium content of atheromatous plaques, although it did not change medial calcium deposition. Vascular calcification is a prominent feature of CKD and it is predictive of increased cardiovascular morbidity and mortality (London et al., 2003).

Apolipoprotein E polymorphisms are also known to influence the development and progression of kidney diseases. Some authors have demonstrated that the ε4 allele has a renoprotective effect in both patients with type 1 and type 2 diabetes (Werle et al., 1998; Eto et al., 1995; Kimura et al., 1998; Eto et al., 2002). On the contrary, a 9-year prospective study of type 2 diabetics showed that a subgroup of patients with a faster decline in renal function had an increased prevalence of the apolipoprotein ε4 allele (Lehtinen et al., 2003). The apolipoprotein ε2 allele has been reported to be a positive predictive factor for progression of renal failure in diabetes type 1 (Araki et al., 2000; Chowdury et al., 1998) and patients with the ε2 had lower total cholesterol, higher urinary albumin excretion, lower LDL-cholesterol and increased TGs (including remnant lipoproteins) than patients with the ε4 allele. This increased level of remnant lipoproteins results in an accumulation of cholesteryl esters by human mesangial cells, leading to glomerulosclerosis and nephropathy (Eto et al., 1995; Eto et al., 2002). As observed, the present results are conflicting and more studies are necessary to better elucidate the exact role of each apoE polymorphism on progression of kidney dysfunction.

Conclusion

Cardiovascular diseases represent a public health care problem worldwide and can be considered the major cause of death among the non-infectious diseases. Particularly, atherosclerosis may lead to several other cardiovascular endpoints, such as myocardial infarction, stroke and peripheral artery disease. Atherosclerosis also is closely related with the development of renal diseases and is the major cause of mortality and morbidity in diabetic patients.

The main risk factor to initiate atherosclerosis is hyperlipidemia. In this context, studies have focused in role of apolipoproteins in the lipid transport disorders and its consequences to the development of several diseases. In this review we highlighted the participation of apolipoprotein E in atherosclerosis, diabetes and renal diseases. The presented data demonstrate that changes in apoE functioning have profound effects on lipid profile, contributing to both the beginning and the progression of these pathologies. Although the main mechanism by which apoE dysfunction contributes to these diseases is the increase in plasma cholesterol levels, we may not rule out the effects of apoE itself, since studies have demonstrated that this protein is required to normal vascular homeostasis.

Among the available experimental models, the apoE knockout mouse appears as a suitable tool for the studies concerning the mechanisms involved in atherogenesis and the interaction between environmental and genetic factors predisposing to atherosclerosis, diabetes and kidney diseases.

References

Anoop S, Misra A, Meena K, Luthra K. Apolipoprotein E polymorphism in cerebrovascular and coronary heart diseases. *Indian Journal of Medical Research*. 2010; 132: p. 363-378.

Araki S, Moczulski DK, Hanna L, Scott LJ, Warram JH, Krolewski AS. APOE polymorphisms and the development of diabetic nephropathy in type 1 diabetes: results of case-control and family-based studies. *Diabetes*. 2000; 49(12): p. 2190-2195.

Arbones-Mainar JM, Johnson LA, Altenburg MK, Maeda N. Differential modulation of diet-induced obesity and adipocyte functionality by human apolipoprotein E3 and E4 in mice. *International Journal of Obesity*. 2008; 32(10): p. 1595-1605.

Atkins RC, Zimmet P. Diabetic kidney disease: act now or pay later. Nature Reviews. *Nephrology*. 2010; 6(3): p. 134-136.

Bachorik PS, Denke MA, Stein EA, Rifkind BM. Lipids and Dyslipoproteinemias. In Henry JB. Clinical Diagnosis and Management by Laboratory Methods. Philadelphia, Pennsylvania: Saunders Company; 2008; p. 259-287.

Balarini CM, Oliveira MZ, Pereira TM, Silva NF, Vasquez EC, Meyrelles SS, Gava AL. Hypercholesterolemia promotes early renal dysfunction in apolipoprotein E-deficient mice. *Lipids in Health and Disease*. 2011; 10: 220.

Banskota NK, Taub R, Zellner K, King GL. Insulin, insulin- like growth factor I and platelet-derived growth factor interact additively in the induction of the protooncogene c- myc and cellular proliferation in cultured bovine aortic smooth muscle cells. *Molecular Endocrinology*. 1989; 3(8): p. 1183-1190.

Bonomini F, Filippini F, Hayek T, Aviram M, Keidar S, Rodella LF, Coleman R, Rezzani R. Apolipoprotein E and its role in aging and survival. *Experimental Gerontology*. 2010; 45(2): p. 149-157.

Boumendjel R, Papari M, Gonzalez M. A rare case of lipoprotein glomerulopathy in a white man: an emerging entity in Asia, rare in the white population. *Archives of Pathology and Laboratory Medicine*. 2010; 134(2): p. 279-282.

Bruneval P, Bariéty J, Bélair MF, Mandet C, Heudes D, Nicoletti A. Mesangial expansion associated with glomerular endothelial cell activation and macrophage recruitment is developing in hyperlipidaemic apoE null mice. *Nephrology, Dialysis, Transplantation*. 2002; 17(12): p. 2099-2107.

Calkin AC, Allen TJ. Diabetes Mellitus-Associated Atherosclerosis: Mechanisms Involved and Potential for Pharmacological Invention. *American Journal of Cardiovascular Drugs*. 2006; 6(1): p. 15-40.

Calkin AC, Giunti S, Sheehy KJ, Chew C, Boolell V, Rajaram YS, Cooper ME, Jandeleit-Dahm KA. The HMG-CoA reductase inhibitor rosuvastatin and the angiotensin receptor antagonist candesartan attenuate atherosclerosis in an apolipoprotein E-deficient mouse model of diabetes via effects on advanced glycation, oxidative stress and inflammation. *Diabetologia*. 2008; 51(9): p. 1731-1740.

Candido R, Allen TJ, Lassila M, Cao Z, Thallas V, Cooper ME, Jandeleit-Dahm KA. Irbesartan but Not Amlodipine Suppresses Diabetes-Associated Atherosclerosis. *Circulation*. 2004; 109(12): p. 1536-1542.

Candido R, Jandeleit-Dahm KA, Cao Z, Nesteroff SP, Burns WC, Twigg SM, Dilley RJ, Cooper ME, Allen TJ. Prevention of Accelerated Atherosclerosis by Angiotensin-Converting Enzyme Inhibition in Diabetic Apolipoprotein E–Deficient Mice. *Circulation*. 2002; 106(2): p. 246-253.

Cardillo C, Nambi SS, Kilcoyne CM, Choucair WK, Katz A, Quon MJ, Panza JA. Insulin stimulates both endothelin and nitric oxide activity in the human forearm. *Circulation*. 1999; 100(8): p. 820-825.

Chaudhary R, Likidlilid A, Peerapatdit T, Tresukosol D, Srisuma S, Ratanamaneechat S, Sriratanasathavorn C. Apolipoprotein E gene polymorphism: effects on plasma lipids and risk of type 2 diabetes and coronary artery disease. *Cardiovascular Diabetology*. 2012; 11(1): 36.

Chen G, Paka L, Kako Y, Singhal P, Duan W, Pillarisetti S. A Protective Role for Kidney Apolipoprotein E: Regulation of Mesangial Cell Proliferation and Matrix Expansion. *The Journal of Biological Chemistry*. 2001; 276(52): p. 49142-49147.

Chowdhury TA, Dyer PH, Kumar S, Gibson SP, Rowe BR, Davies SJ, Marshall SM, Morris PJ, Gill GV, Feeney S, Maxwell P, Savage D, Boulton AJ, Todd JA, Dunger D, Barnett AH, Bain SC. Association of apolipoprotein epsilon2 allele with diabetic nephropathy in Caucasian subjects with IDDM. *Diabetes*. 1998; 47(2): p. 278-280.

Dart A, Sherrard B, Simpson H. Influence of apo E phenotype on postprandial triglyceride and glucose responses in subjects with and without coronary heart disease. *Atherosclerosis*. 1997; 130: p. 161-170.

Davignon J, Gregg RE, Sing CF. Apolipoprotein E Polymorphism and Atherosclerosis. *Arteriosclerosis*. 1988; 8: p. 1-21.

Dentelli P, Rosso A, Zeoli A, Gambino R, Pegoraro L, Pagano G, Falcioni R, Brizzi MF. Oxidative stress-mediated mesangial cell proliferation requires RAC-1/reactive oxygen species production and beta4 integrin expression. *The Journal of Biological Chemistry*. 2007; 282(36): p. 26101-26110.

Diamond JR. Analogous pathobiologic mechanisms in glomerulosclerosis and atherosclerosis. *Kidney International. Supplement*. 1991; 31: p. 29-34.

Dominiczak MH, Caslake MJ. Apolipoproteins: metabolic role and clinical biochemistry aplications. *Annals of Clinical Biochemistry*. 2011; 48: p. 498-515.

D'Souza A, Hussain M, Howarth FC, Woods NM, Bidasee K, Singh J. Pathogenesis and pathophysiology of accelerated atherosclerosis in the diabetic heart. *Molecular and Cellular Biochemistry*. 2009; 331: p. 89-116.

Eichner JE, Dunn T, Perveen G, Thompson DM, Stewart KE, Stroehla BC. Apolipoprotein E Polymorphism and Cardiovascular Disease: A HuGE Review. *American Journal of Epidemiology*. 2002; 155(6): p. 487-495.

Elosua R, Demissie S, Cupples LA, Meigs JB, Wilson PW, Schaefer EJ, Corella D, Ordovas JM. Obesity modulates the association among APOE genotype, insulin, and glucose in men. *Obesity Research*. 2003; 11(12): p. 1502-1508.

Elosua R, Ordovas JM, Cupples LA, Fox CS, Polak JF, Wolf PA, D'Agostino RA Sr, O'Donnell CJ. Association of APOE genotype with carotid atherosclerosis in men and women: the Framingham Heart Study. *Journal of Lipid Research*. 2004; 45(10): p. 1868-1875.

Elshourbagy NA, Liao WS, Mahley RW, Taylor JM. Apolipoprotein E mRNA is abundant in the brain and adrenals, as well as in the liver, and is present in other periferal tissues of rats and marmosets. *Proceedings of the National Academy of Sciences of the United States of America*. 1985; 82(1): p. 203-207.

Eto M, Horita K, Morikawa A, Nakata H, Okada M, Saito M, Nomura M, Abiko A, Iwashima Y, Ikoda A, et al. Increased frequency of apolipoprotein epsilon 2 allele in non-insulin dependent diabetic (NIDDM) patients with nephropathy. *Clinical Genetics*. 1995; 48(6): p. 288-292.

Eto M, Saito M, Okada M, Kume Y, Kawasaki F, Matsuda M, Yoneda M, Matsuki M, Takigami S, Kaku K. Apolipoprotein E genetic polymorphism, remnant lipoproteins, and nephropathy in type2 diabetic patients. *American Journal of Kidney Diseases*. 2002; 40(2): p. 243-251.

Freedman BI, Bostrom M, Daeihagh P, Bowden DW. Genetic factors in diabetic nephropathy. *Clinical Journal of the American Society of Nephrology*. 2007; 2(6): p. 1306-1316.

Gerrity RG. The Role of the Monocyte in Atherogenesis. I. Transition of Blood-Borne Monocytes Into Foam Cells in Fatty Lesions. *The American Journal of Pathology*. 1981; 103(2): p. 181-190.

Godin DV, Dahlman DM. Effects of hypercholesterolemia on tissue antioxidant status in two species differing in susceptibility to atherosclerosis. *Research Communications in Chemical Pathology and Pharmacology*. 1993; 79(2): p. 151-166.

Goldberg IJ. Clinical review 124: Diabetic dyslipidemia: causes and consequences. *The Journal of Clinical Endocrinology and Metabolism*. 2001; 86: p. 965-971.

Goraya TY, Leibson CL, Palumbo PJ, Weston SA, Killian JM, Pfeifer EA, Jacobsen SJ, Frye RL, Roger VL. Coronary Atherosclerosis in Diabetes Mellitus: A Population-Based Autopsy Study. *Journal of the American College of Cardiology*. 2002; 40(5): p. 946-953.

Greenow K, Pearce NJ, Ramji DP. The key role of apolipoprotein E in atheroscleosis. *Journal of Molecular Medicine*. 2005; 83: p. 329-342.

Grenett HE, Benza RL, Fless GM, Li XN, Davis GC, Booyse FM. Genotype- specific transcriptional regulation of PAI-1 gene by insulin, hypertriglyceridemic VLDL, and Lp (a) in transfected, cultured human endothelial cells. *Arteriosclerosis, Thrombosis, and Vascular Biology*. 1998; 18(11): p. 1803-1809.

Grond J, van Goor H, Erkelens DW, Elema JD. Glomerular sclerotic lesions in the rat. Histochemical analysis of their macromolecular and cellular composition. Virchows Archiv. *B Cell Pathology Including Molecular Pathology*. 1986; 51(6): p. 521-534.

Guang-da X, You-ying L, Zhi-song C, Yu-sheng H, Xiang-jiu Y. Apolipoprotein e4 allele is predictor of coronary artery disease death in elderly patients with type 2 diabetes mellitus. *Atherosclerosis*. 2004; 175(1): p. 77-81.

Haffer SM, Lehto S, Rönnemaa T, Pyörälä K, Laakso M. Mortality from coronary heart disease in subjects with type 2 diabetes and nondiabetic subjects with and without prior myocardial infaction. *The New England Journal of Medicine*. 1998; 339(4): p. 229-234.

Hauser PS, Narayanaswami V, Ryan RO. Apolipoprotein E: from lipid transport to neurobiology. *Progress in Lipid Research*. 2011; 50(1): p. 62-74.

Huang Y. Mechanisms linking apolipoprotein E isoforms with cardiovascular and neurological diseases. *Current Opinion in Lipidology*. 2010; 21: p. 337-345.

Hui DY, Innerarity TL, Milne RW, Marcel YL, Mahley RW. Binding of Chylomicron Remnants and β-Very Low Density Lipoproteins to Hepatic and Extrahepatic Lipoprotein Receptors. A Process Independent of Apolipoprotein B48. *The Journal of Biological Chemistry*. 1984; 259(24): p. 15060-15068.

Innerarity TL, Weisgraber KH, Arnold KS, Rall SC Jr, Mahley RW. Normalization of receptor binding of apolipoprotein E2. Evidence for modulation of the binding site conformation. *The Journal of Biological Chemistry*. 1984; 259(11): p. 7261-7267.

Ivanovski O, Szumilak D, Nguyen-Khoa T, Nikolov IG, Joki N, Mothu N, Maizel J, Westenfeld R, Ketteler M, Lacour B, Drüeke TB, Massy ZA. Effect of Simvastatin in Apolipoprotein E Deficient Mice With Surgically Induced Chronic Renal Failure. *The Journal of Urology*. 2008; 179(4): p. 1631-1636.

Jawien J, Nastalek P, Korbut R. Mouse Models of Experimental Atherosclerosis. *Journal of Physiology and Pharmacology*. 2004; 55(3): p. 503-517.

Kako Y, Massé M, Huang LS, Tall AR, Goldberg IJ. Lipoprotein lipase deficiency and CETP in streptozotocin-treated apoB-expressing mice. *Journal of Lipid Research*. 2002; 43(6): p. 872–877.

Kharbanda R, MacAllister RJ. The Atherosclerosis Time-Line and the Role of Endothelium. *Current Medical Chemistry - Immunology, Endocrine and Metabolic Agents*. 2005; 5: p. 47-52.

Kimura H, Suzuki Y, Gejyo F, Karasawa R, Miyazaki R, Suzuki S, Arakawa M. Apolipoprotein E4 reduces risk of diabetic nephropathy in patients with NIDDM. *American Journal of Kidney Diseases*. 1998; 31(4): p. 666-673.

Kolovou G, Anagnostopoulou K, Mikhailidis DP, Cokkinos DV. Apolipoprotein E Knockout Models. *Current Pharmaceutical Design*. 2008; 14: p. 338-351.

Lalazar A, Weisgraber KH, Rall SC Jr, Giladi H, Innerarity TL, Levanon AZ, Boyles JK, Amit B, Gorecki M, Mahley RW et al. Site-specific mutagenesis of human apolipoprotein E. Receptor binding activity of variants with single amino acid substitution. *The Journal of Biological Chemistry*. 1988; 263(8): p. 3542-3545.

Lehtinen S, Rantalaiho V, Wirta O, Pasternack A, Laippala P, Koivula T, Lehtimäki T. Apolipoprotein E gene polymorphism, hypercholesterolemia and glomerular filtration rate in type 2 diabetic subjects: a 9-year follow-up study. *Journal of Biomedical Science*. 2003; 10(2): p. 260-265.

Li X, Liu Y, Zhang H, Ren L, Li Q, Li N. Animal models for the atherosclerosis research: a review. Protein Cell. 2011a; 2(3): p. 189-201.

Li J, Wang Q, Chai W, Chen MH, Liu Z, Shi W. Hyperglycemia in apolipoprotein E-deficient mouse strains with different atherosclerosis susceptibility. *Cardiovascular Diabetology*. 2011b; 10: p. 117-127.

Libby P. Inflammation in atherosclerosis. *Nature*. 2002; 420: p. 868-874.

Libby P, Okamoto Y, Rocha VZ, Folco E. Inflammation in Atherosclerosis: Transition From Theory to Practice. *Circulation Journal*. 2010; 74: p. 213-220.

Libby P, Ridker PM, Hansson GK. Progress and challenges in translating the biology of atherosclerosis. *Nature*. 2011; 473: p. 317-325.

Lin CT, Xu YF, Wu JY, Chan L. Immunoreactive apolipoprotein E is a widely distributed cellular protein. Immunohistochemical localization of apolipoprotein E in baboon tissues. *The Journal of Clinical Investigation*. 1986; 78(4): p. 947-958.

London GM, Guérin AP, Marchais SJ, Métivier F, Pannier B, Adda H. Arterial media calcification in end-stage renal disease: impact on all-cause and cardiovascular mortality. *Nephrology, Dialysis, Transplantation*. 2003; 18(9): p. 1731-1740.

Lusis AJ. Atherosclerosis. *Nature*. 2000; 407(6801): p. 233-241.

Magoori K, Kang MJ, Ito MR, Kakuuchi H, Ioka RX, Kamataki A, Kim DH, Asaba H, Iwasaki S, Takei YA, Sasaki M, Usui S, Okazaki M, Takahashi S, Ono M, Nose M, Sakai J, Fujino T, Yamamoto TT. Severe hypercholesterolemia, impaired fat tolerance, and advanced atherosclerosis in mice lacking both low density lipoprotein receptor-related protein 5 and apolipoprotein E. *The Journal of Biological Chemistry*. 2003; 278(13): p. 11331-11336.

Mahley RW. Apolipoprotein E: Cholesterol Transport Protein with Expanding Role in Cell Biology. *Science*. 1988; 240: p. 622-630.

Mahley RW, Rall SCJ. Apolipoprotein E: Far More Than a Lipid Transport Protein. *Annual Review of Genomics and Human Genetics*. 2000; 01: p. 507-537.

Meir KS, Leitersdorf E. Atherosclerosis in the Apolipoprotein E-Deficient Mouse: A Decade of Progress. *Arteriosclerosis, Thrombosis, and Vascular Biology*. 2004; 24: p. 1006-1014.

Meyrelles SS, Peotta VA, Pereira TM, Vasquez EC. Endothelial Dysfunction in the Apolipoprotein E-deficient Mouse: insights into the influence of diet, gender and aging. *Lipids in Health and Disease*. 2011; 10: 211.

Moore KJ, Kunjathoor VV, Koehn SL, Manning JJ, Tseng AA, Silver JM, McKee M, Freeman MW. Loss of receptor-mediated lipid uptake via scavenger receptor A or CD36 pathways does not ameliorate atherosclerosis in hyperlipidemic mice. *The Journal of Clinical Investigation*. 2005; 115(8): p. 2192-2201.

Nakashima Y, Plump AS, Raines EW, Breslow JL, Ross R. ApoE-deficient mice develop lesions of all phases of atherosclerosis throughout the arterial tree. *Arteriosclerosis, Thrombosis, and Vascular Biology*. 1994; 14: p. 133-140.

Nordt TK, Sawa H, Fujii S, Bode C, Sobel BE. Augmentation of arterial endothelial cell expression of the plasminogen activator inhibitor type-1 (PAI-1) gene by proinsulin and insulin in vivo. *Journal of Molecular and Cellular Cardiology*. 1998; 30(8): p. 1535-1543.

Oliver FJ, de la Rubia G, Feener EP, Lee ME, Loeken MR, Shiba T, Quertermous T, King GL. Stimulation of endothelin-1 gene expression by insulin in endothelial cells. *The Journal of Biological Chemistry*. 1991; 266(34): p. 23251-23256.

Olivieri O, Martinelli N, Bassi A, Trabetti E, Girelli D, Pizzolo F, Friso S, Pignatti PF, Corrocher R. ApoE epsilon2/epsilon3/epsilon4 polymorphism, ApoC-III/ApoE ratio and metabolic syndrome. *Clinical and Experimental Medicine*. 2007; 7(4): p. 164-172.

Packard RRS, Libby P. Inflammation in Atherosclerosis: From Vascular Biology to Biomarker Discovery and Risk Prediction. *Clinical Chemistry*. 2008; 54(1): p. 24-38.

Park L, Raman KG, Lee KJ, Lu Y, Ferran LJ Jr, Chow WS, Stern D, Schmidt AM . Suppression of accelerated diabetic atherosclerosis by the soluble receptor for advanced glycation endproducts. *Nature Medicine*. 1998; 4(9): p. 1025-1031.

Pedersen TR, Kjekshus J, Berg K, Haghfelt T, Faergeman O, Faergeman G, Pyörälä K, Miettinen T, Wilhelmsen L, Olsson AG, Wedel H; Scandinavian Simvastatin Survival Study Group. Randomised trial of cholesterol lowering in 4444 patients with coronary heart disease: the Scandinavian Simvastatin Survival Study (4S). 1994. *Atherosclerosis. Supplement*. 2004; 5(3): p. 81-87.

Peter R, Cox A, Evans M. Management of diabetes in cardiovascular patients: diabetic heart disease. *Heart*. 2008; 94(3): p. 369-375.

Piedrahita JA, Zhang SH, Hagaman JR, Oliver PM, Maeda N. Generation of mice carrying a mutant apolipoprotein E gene inactivated by gene targeting in embryonic stem cells. *Proceedings of the National Academy of Sciences of the United States of America*. 1992; 89: p. 4471-4475.

Plump AS, Smith JD, Hayek T, Aalto-Setälä K, Walsh A, Verstuyft JG, Rubin RM, Breslow JL. Severe Hypercholesterolemia and Atherosclerosis in Apolipoprotein E-Deficient Mice Created by Homologous Recombination in ES Cells. *Cell*. 1992; 71: p. 343-353.

Rall SCJ, Mahley RW. The role of apolipoprotein E genetic variants in lipoprotein disorders. *Journal of Internal Medicine*. 1992; 231: p. 653-659.

Rask-Madsen C, Buonomo E, Li Q, Park K, Clermont AC, Yerokun O, Rekhter M, King GL. Hyperinsulinemia does not change atherosclerosis development in apolipoprotein e null mice. *Arteriosclerosis, Thrombosis, and Vascular Biology*. 2012; 32(5): p. 1124-1131.

Rask-Madsen C, Li Q, Freund B, Feather D, Abramov R, Wu IH, Chen K, Yamamoto-Hiraoka J, Goldenbogen J, Sotiropoulos KB, Clermont A, Geraldes P, Dall'Osso C, Wagers AJ, Huang PL, Rekhter M, Scalia R, Kahn CR, King GL. Loss of insulin signaling in vascular endothelial cells accelerates atherosclerosis in apolipoprotein E null mice. *Cell Metabolism*. 2010; 11(5): p. 379-389.

Reddick RL, Zhang SH, Maeda N. Atherosclerosis in mice lacking apo E. Evaluation of lesional development and progression. *Arteriosclerosis, Thrombosis, and Vascular Biology*. 1994; 14: p. 141-147.

Rikitake Y, Liao JK. Rho GTPases, statins, and nitric oxide. *Circulation Research*. 2005; 97(12): p. 1232-1235.

Rosenfeld ME, Polinsky P, Virmani R, Kauser K, Rubanyi G, Schwartz SM. Advanced atherosclerotic lesions in the innominate artery of the ApoE knockout mouse. *Arteriosclerosis, Thrombosis, and Vascular Biology*. 2000; 20(12): p. 2587-2592.

Ross R. Atherosclerosis - an inflammatory disease. *New England Journal of Medicine*. 1999; 340(2): p. 115-126.

Schaeffner ES, Kurth T, Curhan GC, Glynn RJ, Rexrode KM, Baigent C, Buring JE, Gaziano JM. Cholesterol and the risk of renal dysfunction in apparently healthy men. *Journal of the American Society of Nephrology*. 2003; 14(8): p. 2084-2091.

Scuteri A, Najjar SS, Muller D, Andres R, Morrell CH, Zonderman AB, Lakatta EG. apoE4 allele and the natural history of cardiovascular risk factors. *American Journal Physiology. Endocrinology and Metabolism*. 2005; 289(2): p. 322-327.

Shimano H, Ohsuga J, Shimada M, Namba Y, Gotoda T, Harada K, Katsuki M, Yazaki Y, Yamada N. Inhibition of diet-induced atheroma formation in transgenic mice expressing apolipoprotein E in the arterial wall. *The Journal of Clinical Investigation.* 1995; 95(2): p. 469-476.

Shore VG, Shore B. Heterogeneity of Human Plasma Very Low Density Lipoproteins. Separation of Species Differing in Protein Components. *Biochemistry.* 1973; 12(3): p. 502-507.

Siest G, Pillot T, Régis-Bailly A, Leininger-Muller B, Steinmetz J, Galteau MM, Visvikis S. Apolipoprotein E: an important gene and protein to follow in laboratory medicine. *Clinical Chemistry.* 1995; 41: p. 1068-1086.

Sima A, Iordan A, Stancu C. Apolipoprotein E polymorphism - a risk factor for metabolic syndrome. *Clinical Chemistry and Laboratory Medicine.* 2007; 45(9): p. 1149-1153.

Simionescu N, Vasile E, Lupu F, Popescu G, Simionescu M. Prelesional events in atherogenesis: accumulation of extracellular cholesterol-rich liposomes in the arterial intima and cardiac valves of the hyperlipidemic rabbit. *The American Journal of Pathology.* 1986; 123(1): p. 109-125.

Sing CF, Davignon J. Role of the apolipoprotein E polymosphism in determining normal plasma lipid and lipoprotein variation. *American Journal of Human Genetics.* 1985; 37: p. 268-285.

Tabas I. Macrophage death and defective inflammation resolution in atherosclerosis. Nature Reviews. Immunology. 2010; 10(1): p. 36-46.

Tsimihodimos V, Elisaf M. Lipoprotein glomerulopathy. *Current Opinion in Lipidology.* 2011; 22: p. 262-269.

Vasquez EC, Peotta VA, Gava AL, Pereira TMC, Meyrelles SS. Cardiac and vascular phenotypes in the apolipoprotein E-deficient mouse. *Journal of Biomedical Science.* 2012; 19: 22.

Vaziri ND, Kim HJ, Moradi H, Farmand F, Navab K, Navab M, Hama S, Fogelman AM, Quiroz Y, Rodriguez-Iturbe B. Amelioration of nephropathy with apoA-1 mimetic peptide in apoE-deficient mice. *Nephrology, dialysis, transplantation.* 2010; 25(11): p. 3525-3534.

Vergès B. Lipid modification in type 2 diabetes: the role of LDL and HDL. *Fundamental and Clinical Pharmacology.* 2009; 23(6): p. 681-685.

Weiner DE, Tabatabai S, Tighiouart H, Elsayed E, Bansal N, Griffith J, Salem DN, Levey AS, Sarnak MJ. Cardiovascular outcomes and all-cause mortality: exploring the interaction between CKD and cardiovascular disease. *American Journal of Kidney Diseases.* 2006; 48(3): p. 392-401.

Weisgraber KH, Rall SCJ, Mahley RW. Human E apoprotein heterogeneity. Cysteine-arginine interchanges in the amino acid sequence of the apo-E isoforms. *The Journal of Biological Chemistry.* 1981; 256: p. 9077-9083.

Wen M, Segerer S, Dantas M, Brown PA, Hudkins KL, Goodpaster T, Kirk E, LeBoeuf RC, Alpers CE. Renal injury in apolipoprotein E-deficient mice. *Laboratory Investigation.* 2002; 82(8): p. 999-1006.

Werle E, Fiehn W, Hasslacher C. Apolipoprotein E polymorphism and renal function in German type 1 and type 2 diabetic patients. *Diabetes Care.* 1998; 21(6): p. 994-998.

World Health Organization. [Online].; 2008 [cited 2012]. Available from: URL "http://www.who.int".

Zhang C, Akira M, Hideki H, Hisashi S, Seikoh H. Very low and intermediate density lipoprotein fractions from apolipoprotein E gene-knockout mice induce cholesteryl ester accumulation in J774 macrophages. *Chinese Medical Journal*. 1999; 112(6): p. 543-545.

Zhang H, Wu LM, Wu J. Cross-Talk between Apolipoprotein E and Cytokines. *Mediators of Inflammation*. 2011; 2011. Epub 2011.

Zhou TB, Qin YH, Lei FY, Su LN, Zhao YJ, Huang WF. ApoE Expression in Glomerulus and Correlation with Glomerulosclerosis Induced by Adriamycin in Rats. *Renal Failure*. 2011a; 33(3): p. 348-354.

Zhou TB, Qin YH, Lei FY, Su LN, Zhao YJ, Huang WF. All-trans retinoic acid regulates the expression of apolipoprotein E in rats with glomerulosclerosis induced by Adriamycin. *Experimental and Molecular Pathology*. 2011b; 90(3): p. 287-294.

In: Apolipoproteins
Editors: A. D. Sidorov and M. Y. Nikitin
ISBN: 978-1-62257-484-1

Chapter IV

Role of Functional Variants and Mutations of the Apolipoprotein A5 Gene in Human Pathology

Balázs Duga, Béla I. Melegh, Katalin Sümegi, Anita Maász, Péter Kisfali, Katalin Komlósi and Béla Melegh

Department of Medical Genetics, University of Pécs;
and Szentágothay Research Center, Pécs, Hungary

Abstract

One of the many factors affecting the lipid metabolism by a complex manner is the apolipoprotein A-5 (ApoA5). The gene of the *ApoA5* is located on chromosome 11q23 in the *ApoA1/C3/A4/A5* gene cluster. With a moderate rage of circulating plasma ApoA5 concentration (50-250 ng/ml), it plays an effective regulatory role in triglyceride metabolism. In the plasma, the protein is found mainly on TG rich lipoproteins such as chylomicrons and VLDL where it shows an opposite effect as the ApoC3, namely enhancing lipoprotein lipase mediated triglyceride catabolism. It comes from this key role of the ApoA5, that the common naturally occurring variants (like T-1131C, T1259C, C56G, and IVS3+G476A) and haplotypes determined by them are associated with elevated plasma triglyceride concentrations, these variants and haplotype combinations have been shown to confer risk or protection for development of cardiovascular disease, stroke and metabolic syndrome. However, there are also some less frequent genetic variants that in combination with the common allelic variants of the gene can define haplotypes that are associated with more pronounced triglyceride level increase. In addition, there are rare mutations of the *ApoA5* gene which are associated with specific complex phenotype that includes extremely high triglyceride levels with multiple organ pathology. The current chapter summarizes these three groups represented by point mutations, deletion/insertion mutations, splicing mutations, and associate with different human pathology.

Discovery of Apolipoprotein A5

Apolipoprotein A5 (ApoA5), a newly identified member of the apoprotein family, which includes well known proteins like ApoA1, ApoA4, ApoC3. ApoA5 was discovered independently by two research teams in 2001, despite the fact that they used two different techniques. One team, van der Vliet et al. was searching for liver regenerating factors with cDNA subtractive hybridization. They found an upregulated and unidentified gene in rat liver six hours after partial hepatectomy. The protein showed some homology to other apoproteins like ApoA1 and ApoA4 [1]. The other team, Pennachio et al. was using comparative genome sequencing between mouse and human DNA, searching for regulator genes in lipid metabolism [2]. They described a gene in the neighbouring area of the *ApoA1/C3/A4* gene cluster on chromosome 11q23, which was located 27 kbp far from 3' end of the *ApoA4* gene. The mature human ApoA5 is a 39 kDa protein, which is expressed exclusively in the liver. According to further studies, the liver produces ApoA5 proteins [3], although a very low plasma concentration was found in humans (0.1-0.4 μg/ml) [4,5], which is 2000-fold lower than ApoC3, meaning that only one in 24 VLDL particles can carry an ApoA5 molecule. This explains the difficulty to discovering this apoprotein [6].

Structure and Molecular Interactions of Apolipoprotein A5

ApoA5 encodes a 366 amino acid residue protein, while mature ApoA5 contains 343 amino acid residues in humans [2]. ApoA5 is a hydrophobic protein, which has an amphipathic α-helix secondary structure; therefore the ApoA5 protein is insoluble at neutral pH in aqueous solution [7,8]. In absence of lipids the N-terminal residues 1-146 form a helix bundle [9]. This fragment region is water soluble contrary to the full length protein [10]. Results show that residues 1-146 can bind to lipoproteins like HDL and VLDL. In the attendance of lipids, ApoA5 shows good solubility due to the lipid binding residues 293-343 at the C-terminal end. Thus, like other lipoproteins, ApoA5 also has an α-helix forming N-terminal domain and a lipid-binding C-terminal domain, although Sun et al. [11] distinguished six different regions in ApoA5 by using secondary structure prediction models [8]. Residues 192–238 are necessary for lipid binding and activation of LPL, but the C-terminal end is not a requisite for ApoA5 to bind a folded secondary structure, as whole deletion mutants' studies were revealed [11]. The principal heparin-binding domain of ApoA5, which contains four positively charged residues (R210, K211, K215, K217), are necessary between ApoA5 and the LPL-anchoring protein (GPIHBP1; Glycosyl-phosphatidylinositol-anchored high density lipoprotein-binding protein 1) interaction [12,13]. ApoA5 has been shown to bind GPIHBP1 in vitro and this interaction has been postulated to facilitate lipoprotein lipase (LPL) mediated hydrolysis of the triglyceride (TG) component of chylomicrons (CM). The positively charged heparin-binding sequence within ApoA5 and the acidic domain in GPIHBP1 are both required for binding [14].

ApoA5 can exist as a disulfide-linked homodimer or can form heterodimers with other apolipoproteins due to the single cystein at residue 204. Studies by Alborn et al. showed that the cysteine sulfhydryl group remains free, indicating that ApoA5 is monomeric in human plasma [15]. Results of the studies show that ApoA5 can connect to heparin and to LDL receptor (LDLr) gene family members (LDLr related protein 1 (LRP1) and the mosaic receptor LR11/SorLA) through a 42 amino acid stretch (residues 186–227), which contains eight Arg/Lys and three His amino acid [8,16,17,18]. As with ApoB and ApoE with LDLr family members and with heparan sulfate proteoglycans (HSPG, the same mechanism of interaction can probably be found in ApoA5, involving positively charged regions in the ligands and negatively charged regions in the receptors. The double mutant Arg210Glu/ Lys211Gln, which shows decreased binding to heparin and LRP1, confirms the importance of the positively charged residues in interaction [8,17]. The N-terminal end of ApoA5 was recently shown to interact with cell surface midkine (neurite growth-promoting factor 2; NEGF2) and to be internalized in pancreatic β-cells, leading to increased insulin secretion [19]. This could be part of the explanation why insulin resistance was seen in *ApoA5* knockout animals [20,8].

Apolipoprotein A5 Mouse Models and Metabolic Experiments

Several studies used human ApoA5 transgenic and ApoA5 deficient mouse models to investigate the lipid metabolic role of apolipoprotein A5. Compared to the wild type controls transgenic mice showed 40% reduced plasma TG, and ApoA5 deficient mice had significantly elevated TG levels, which was approximately four times higher than their wild typed littermates. Fast protein liquid chromatography (FPLC) and gradient gel electrophoresis were used to characterize the lipoprotein particles and revealed differences were found in VLDL levels.

One of the most important questions is raised, whether the ApoA5 effect can take part of ApoC3, which strongly inhibits plasma TG hydrolysis [21]. Results showed that in ApoA5 deficient animals an elevated plasma level of ApoC3 was found, but decreased in ApoA5 transgenic animals [2]. Normal TG level were found in double transgenic and double knockout mice for ApoC3 and ApoA5.

Despite their different plasma levels, this study confirmed the connection between these two apoproteins; they are antagonist for each other [22,23]. The possible interplay between ApoA5 and LPL (lipoprotein lipase), which catalyzes the TG hydrolysis in lipoproteins, was investigated by crossbreeding a human LPL transgenic line with ApoA5 deficient mice and LPL deficient mice with an ApoA5 transgene. As results show, in ApoA5 deficient mouse, the elevated LPL activity completely normalized hypertriglyceridaemia, however, over expression of human ApoA-V influenced TG levels only slightly when LPL was reduced [24,25].

Apolipoprotein A5 Molecular Mechanism and Mode of Action

Three hypotheses explain the mechanism of ApoA5 actions: (1) ApoA5 acts through an intracellular mechanism and is involved in VLDL synthesis and/or secretion. (2) ApoA5 accelerates the hydrolysis of TG-rich lipoproteins by affecting LPL, which could be either direct or via other regulator apolipoproteins such as ApoC3. (3) ApoA5 acts as a ligand to lipoprotein receptors or proteoglycans and therefore promotes receptor-mediated endocytosis of lipoproteins [8].

Data from different studies support the role of ApoA5 in extracellular TG metabolism and there is increasing support for an additional function of ApoA5 as a receptor ligand, thus there is support for all three possible modes of action. Nevertheless, the intracellular role of ApoA5 for lipoprotein assembly and secretion is still more theoretical [8].

Former investigations suggest that ApoA5 can play a role in the reduction of plasma TG via intracellularly on lipoprotein assembly [3]. Further studies show that ApoA5 has a very important function in the TG regulation. ApoA5 may affect for plasma TG level, furthermore it may decrease hepatic VLDL production by binding to lipids and cellular membranes and through this, inhibit VLDL assembly and secretion [3,7]. Several studies' results show that ApoA5 has a TG reducing effect by accelerating plasma TG hydrolysis. The most significant plasma TG level reducing effects of ApoA5 are the acceleration of plasma TG hydrolysis by modulating LPL activity or by amending the effects or the concentrations of other apolipoproteins like ApoC3. ApoC3 is an apolipoprotein, which has a physiological antagonist effect for the LPL activity unlike ApoA5 [22]. Since, ApoA5 can change the effect or the concentration of ApoC3, it can modify the plasma TG level.

ApoA5 can be found mostly on the surface of VLDL or HDL lipoproteins [24]. When the VLDL/CM-ApoA5 complex reaches the endothelium, it connects to the GPIHBP1 protein or HSPG, which is anchored to the endothelium, and to the LPLs. The LPLs can be found in dimeric form on the GPIHBP1 protein or HSPG surface and catalysing the lipoprotein TG hydrolysis. Based on several studies, researchers assume that ApoA5 may influence TG hydrolysis in different ways. This depends on the anchoring molecule, which can be HSPG or GPIHBP1 [13]. If the VLDL/CM-ApoA5 complex connects to the HSPG molecule, this interaction can assist ApoC-2 activation of LPL, resulting in increased speed of TG hydrolysis. After the catabolism of TG-reach lipoproteins (VLDL or chylomicron (CM)), ApoA5 exfoliates from the remnant particle and transfer to nascent HDL. Furthermore ApoA5 can bind to the GPIHBP1 homodimer and LPLs, where the interaction may accelerate the TG hydrolysis in CM/VLDL. Furthermore, ApoA5 can interact with LPLR family members and induces endocytosis of remnant lipoproteins. Nevertheless, the exact mechanisms of ApoA5 have not been elucidated yet.

Common Polymorphisms in *Apoa5*

Apolipoprotein gene cluster *ApoA1/C3/A4/A5* on chromosome 11q23 plays a pivotal role in TG metabolism, and apolipoprotein A5 (ApoA5) has emerged as an important modulator of serum TG concentration [2, 26, 27].

In the past few years, researchers could identify several polymorphisms in *ApoA5* gene. Only some of them cause elevated TG levels alone or with other polymorphisms in a haplogroup [28]. Four single nucleotide polymorphisms (SNP) were identified in the *ApoA5* gene at the very beginning, which were the g.-1131T>C (rs662799) in the promoter region, the g.1259T>C (rs2266788) in the 3' untranslated region (UTR), the c.56C>G (p.Ser19Trp, rs3135506) in the third exon and the g.IVS3+476G>A (rs2072560) in the third intron. Three of these SNPs cause 50% higher TG levels in heterozygous state, than in patients who were homozygous for the major allele [2]. Epidemiological and clinical studies show that increased (TG) concentrations are an independent risk factor for coronary artery disease (CAD) [27, 29, 30].

g.-1131T>C (rs662799)

The g.-1131T>C variant in the promoter region is the most extensively studied among the naturally occurring variants of *ApoA5* gene. The alteration was found in 6% of the healthy European population. The frequency of the variant is very different among other populations: 30% of the Japanese, 27% the Chinese and 20% of the Indian population carried the mutant allele [HapMap] [31]. Several studies examined this *ApoA5* polymorphism minor allele effect for the TG level and the risk of diseases development. Results suggest that the minor C allele of the *ApoA5* T-1131C polymorphism has been shown associated with the increased TG level and through this, may affect the emergence of several diseases, like coronary artery disease (CAD), metabolic syndrome and stroke [32,33,34].

Nevertheless, recent data support a connection [23,35-40], although earlier studies did not showed correlation between the *ApoA5* polymorphisms and TG concentrations [4,39]. The -1131C allele was associated with plasma TG, but not with the ApoA5 concentration as Northwick Park Heart Study II showed [37]. *ApoA5* T-1131C polymorphism was also investigated in a northern Chinese Han population, where the results confirmed that the minor allele was associated with increased serum TG levels [41]. Furthermore Japanese, German and Austrian studies examined the same *ApoA5* T-1131C polymorphism; while the Japanese researchers could detect association, until the German-Austrian study could not observe any association between the minor allele of the T-1131C and the higher plasma TG levels. Pennacchio et al. also found an association between T-1131C polymorphism and plasma TG level. Studies showed that patients, who suffer from these diseases like metabolic syndrome, CVD or stroke, have elevated TG level contrary to the control group and the -1131C incidence rate in patients is much higher [42]. Arnedo et al. examined the effect T-1131C of the plasma TG level and the role of the disease development [43].

These results suggest that -1131C is a risk factor for elevated TG level and through this it may have an important role in the emergence diseases. Despite the lack of association between CVD and ApoA5 concentration has an importance in the pathogenesis of dyslipidemia and CVD [39]. The minor -1131C polymorphism allele has an elevated risk for CAD, despite the fact that the plasma level of ApoA5 is not related with CAD. -1131C can increase the TG level as several study proved. The elevated TG level can also be a trigger for developing CAD, metabolic syndrome and stroke [39,44-47].

g.IVS3+476G>A (rs2072560)

Another major polymorphism is IVS3+G476A, which is located in the third intron of the *ApoA5* gene. Studies found that the minor allele of IVS3+G476A variant has a TG increasing effect, as it was in the case in T-1131C. Although, the IVS3+G476A is an intronic polymorphism of *ApoA5*, it can influence the function of the protein transcript, which can secondarily modify the interaction of ApoA5 with the lipoprotein lipase and ultimately results in increasing the circulating TG levels [2,48-50]. Numerous studies examined the IVS3+G476A polymorphism, and its effect on disease development. Results suggest that the IVS3+G476A polymorphism has a massive ability to elevate the TG level, which can be a risk factor for CAD, metabolic syndrome, and stroke [50].

In the Hungarian population the allele frequency of IVS3+G476A was significantly higher in metabolic syndrome patients compared to controls. Multiple regression analysis revealed that carrying the IVS3+G476A allelic variant is an increased risk for developing metabolic syndrome [51]. Further studies showed that the IVS3+476A allele was more frequent in all stroke subgroups compared to controls. Multiple regression analysis revealed that IVS3+476A allele represents an independent risk factor for stroke [50].

g.1259T>C (rs2266788)

Relatively small amount of imformation is available about the variant in 3'-untranslated (3'-UTR) region of *ApoA5* gene compared to other variants. The T1259C was examined together with the other *ApoA5* polymorphisms (T-1131C; IVS3+G476A; C56G). Results show that the T1259C minor C allele can cause elevated TG levels. Despite the fact that T1259C may cause an elevated TG level in people who carry the 1259C minor allele, an association for the development of cerebrovascular diseases and metabolic syndrome was not found, contrary to the IVS3+476A allele [51,50].

c.56C>G (p.Ser19Trp, rs3135506)

C56G is localized in the coding region, which is in the third exon in the *ApoA5* gene. Since it is in the coding region, it may change the structure of the protein. C56G is also known as S19W, which means that 19th amino acid in the ApoA5 is hydrophilic serine (Ser) and changes to hydrophobic tryptophan (Trp). The alteration was found in less than 0.1% of the Japanese and Chinese populations. Additionally, 3, 4.8, 4.8 and 15% of the Indian, Afro-American, French and Spanish population carry the c.56C>G variants, respectively [28,52] (HapMap).

Several studies reveal that C56G minor allele may be associated with elevated TG level. Maasz et al. [53] reported that G allele of *ApoA5* C56G is a higher risk for the development of large-vessel-associated ischemic stroke. In both males and females the Trp19 carriers have significantly higher TG levels compared to the Ser19 homozygous individuals [47]. As expected, the frequencies of the carriers of the less common allele Trp19 are more than twice higher in hypertriglyceridemic patients than in control population [44]. Moreover, the minor G allele of c.56C>G SNP was associated with an approximately 50% higher risk for metabolic syndrome [39].

Haplotypes

Not only simple SNPs can cause elevated TG levels, but also haplotypes. A set of SNPs located on the same chromosome create a haplotype, and they are statistically in linkage. These SNPs in a proper haplotype can cause higher TG levels, contrary to one SNP.

Table 1. Major haplotypes of Apolipoprotein A5

Haplotypes	*T-1131C*	*IVS3+ G476A*	*T1259C*	*C56G*
*ApoA5*1*	T	G	T	C
*ApoA5*2*	C	A	C	C
*ApoA5*3*	T	G	T	G
*ApoA5*4*	C	G	T	C
*ApoA5*5*	T	G	C	C

Pennacchio et al. confirmed that the most common alterations in the *ApoA5* gene are in strong linkage disequilibrium and constitute two major haplotype variant: ApoA5*2 (-1131C, 1259C, IVS3+476A) and ApoA5*3 (56G). These two haplotypes together with wild type haplotype (ApoA5*1,*2,*3) account for approximately 98% of all haplotypes in the average populations [28]. The remaining 2% includes rare haplotype variants like ApoA5*4 (-1131C) and ApoA5*5 (1259C) [Table 1.]. Four of five SNPs have already been published, but ApoA5*5 has not been reported yet.

Significantly elevated serum TG levels were found in association with the ApoA5*2 haplotype in metabolic syndrome and in a control group by Kisfali et al. While an approximately 2.7-fold accumulation of the ApoA5*2 haplotype could be observed in the metabolic syndrome group, the prevalence of the ApoA5*5 was 5.3-times less in the metabolic syndrome patients compared to controls [33].

Logistic regression analysis revealed that the ApoA5*2 haplotype confers significant susceptibility for the development of metabolic syndrome. Results of the logistic regression analysis suggested that in contrast to the ApoA5*2, the ApoA5*5 haplotype might have an independent protective effect against metabolic syndrome [33].

In another haplotype study [54], the major haplotype tagging SNPs and the major haplotypes were compared in paediatric obese children (n = 232) with normal controls (n = 137). The ApoA5*2 haplotype was found to confer to risk for development of obesity, while ApoA5*4, which composed by the -1131C variant alone, did not.

The main message is, similar to the previous paper [33] that haplotype analysis must be done instead of just the SNP test, since -1131C susceptibility was limitedted only to one single haplotype.

Naturally Occurring Rare Functional Variants and Mutations

Besides the common naturally occurring variants of the gene and their natural major haplotypes are known to associate with moderately elevated TG levels, and also are known to confer risk or protection for major polygenic diseases, like coronary heart disease, stroke, or metabolic syndrome, as discussed earlier in this chapter. Soon after the recognition of these associations, there were indications suggesting that there are also some less frequent genetic variants that in combination with the common allelic variants of the gene can define haplotypes that are associated with more pronounced TG level increase.

In addition, it became evident soon in the ApoA5 research, that there are rare mutations of the *ApoA5* gene which are associated with specific complex phenotypes and different types of hyperlipoproteinemias, which can include extremely high TG levels with multiple organ pathology. These rare mutations may cause inheritable hypertriglyceridemia (HTG), but they are presented such a low frequency that they could not be captured by genotyping arrays. The identification of new mutations is linked to the sequencing the *ApoA5* gene of patients with HTG with an unusual pattern, or by huge resequencing studies.

Severe HTG is a general condition associated with different pathological phenotypes including different lipoproteinemias and has a few well-documented genetic contributors, including lipoprotein lipase, ApoC2, ApoE, and environmental factors such as diet or life style [2,55]. Hyperlipoproteinemia type I and type V both involve HTG with high levels on fasting chylomicron levels. In Type V VLDL fraction levels are also high [55]. In dysbetalipoproteinaemia (hyperlipoproteinaemia type III) HTG is associated with increased levels of TG-rich lipoprotein remnants, this disease is usually caused by a defective ApoE2 isoform [56].

The *ApoA5* gene's first pathogenic mutation was discovered in 2005 by Oliva et al [57]. The proband was a 9-year old boy with severe HTG (over 50mmol/L) and anamnestic data of abdominal pain, xanthomas and mild hepatosplenomegaly. His phenotype was described as Type I hyperlipoproteinaemia but LPL and ApoC2 mutations were excluded. After sequencing the *ApoA5* gene, he was found to be homozygous for a nucletotid in exon four [57] resulting finally in a Q148X nonsense mutation. The mutation caused premature termination of transcription and a reduced sized defective protein.

The patient was found to have complete *ApoA5* deficiency as no ApoA5 could be detected in his plasma. Further examination of the family showed that heterozygous carriers required additional genetic or environmental factors for development of HTG. All carriers of this mutation shared the common variant p.S19W described by Talmud et al [58], but the link between the mutation and the polymorphism is not clear yet. Olivia et al. defined this mutation as recessive. The patients-HTG was successfully reduced with ω-3 fatty acid supplementation.

The second mutation was discovered in the same year by Marcia et al [59]. ApoA5 was studied in a family with history of unusual, late onset hyperchylomicronemia described as type V hyperlipoproteinemia with vertical transmission. After excluding LPL and ApoC2 as the genetic background of the symptoms they sequenced the *ApoA5* gene finding a mutation on the c.415 position where the wild cytosine was changed for a thymidine. The mutation Q139X creates a premature truncation and thus results in ApoA5 mediated LPL defect leading to lipolysis impairment. All members of the family with severe HTG were either homozygote for the mutation or heterozygote plus carriers of the known TG level raiser ApoA5*2 or ApoA5*3 haplotype.

The third mutation was found in a 17 year-old male by Olivia el al [60]. The proband had HTG (5-12mmol/L), low HDL-C levels (below 1mmol/L) and eruptive xanthomas suggesting chylomicronaemia syndrome. His LPL activity was normal and no mutations were found in the LPL or the *ApoC2* genes. After sequencing the *ApoA5* gene the patient was found to be homozygous for a point mutation at the c.289 position. The nucleotide change created a nonsense mutation (p.Q97X). No ApoA5 was detectable in the patient plasma showing complete *ApoA5* deficiency. He was also homozygous for the common allele in the promoter of the *ApoA5* gene (-482C/C). The other interesting find in the patient was the persistently low level of plasma HDL-C, which, unlike his TG level was only marginally affected by ω-3 fatty acid supplementation. The hypothesis that the absence of ApoA5, which is a minor component of HDL, makes HDL more unstable and more easily removed from the circulation, is unlikely according to the very low concentration of ApoA5. It is more likely that the delayed TG hydrolysis, due to ApoA5 deficiency is related to the increased level of ApoC3 (an inhibitor of LPL) [61], and reduces the availability of surface components of TG-rich lipoproteins, which contribute to HDL formation. Recent studies showed that adenovirus mediated delivery of *ApoA5* into HTG *ApoC3* transgenic mice not only reduced TG and VLDL-C level but also increased HDL-C level with an increase of both the number and size of HDL particles [62]. These data suggest that in addition to its TG-lowering effects, ApoA5 plays an important role in modulating HDL maturation and cholesterol metabolism.

In 2008, Dorfmeister et al. [63] performed a study aimed to identify rare ApoA5 variant in 130 patients with severe HTG via sequencing the *ApoA5* gene. They identified three novel missense mutations: p.E255G, p.G271C and p.H321L. The first mutation p.E255G (c.764A>G) was identified in a 32 year-old female who had pregnancy related Type I hyperlipoproteinemia. She was also heterozygous for the common ApoA5 p.S19Wpoly-morphism and homozygous for LPL p.W86G, which variation was previously reported in a pediatric Type I hyperlipoproteinemia [64]. During her pregnancies she developed serum TG level over 75mmol/L and cutaneous xanthomas, but was asymptomatic when not pregnant. The second p.G271C (c.821G>T) mutation was found in a heterozygous form in a 43 year-old female who had persistent HTG (20mmol/L), and multiple cases of pancreatitis. The proband was also homozygous for the common g.-1131T>C variant and surprisingly plasma ApoA5 level was 15 times higher than the mean level in normo-lipidemic controls. The third p.H321L (c.962A>T) uncommon variant was identified in a 46 year old male who was also heterozygous for p.S19W. His plasma TG level was over 63mmol/L and the patient suffered from acute pancreatitis. Molecular modeling methods suggested that these novel mutations change ApoA5 in a way that its ability to interact with LPL is reduced.

Recently, genome wide association studies (GWAS) were also used to identify candidate variants in a cohort of patient with HTG. Johansen et al. [65] designed a study including a total of 555 individuals with HTG and 1,319 controls in two cohorts of the study: the GWAS cohort included 463 HTG patients and 1,197 controls, and the sequencing cohort included 438 affected individuals and 327 controls. They found several new sequence alterations from which p.N66S was novel and exclusive to affected individuals. They also found 3 mutations with proven biological dysfunction or truncation: p.G185C, p.Q305X and p.D332Vfs336X, from which p.G185C was previously identified in 2003 by Kao et al. [66] who described the nucleotide change as a common polymorphism, however according to Polyphen analysis the variant is probably deleterious.

Table 2. Point mutations of Apolipoprotein A5

Mutation	TG	Associated variants	Clinical relevance	Ref
Q148X(c.442C>T)	extreme(50mmol/L)	S19W, heterozygous for Apo C3 -482 C/T polymorphism APOA5*2APOA5*3 haplotype	abdominal pain , xanthomas, hyperchylomicronemia	[57]
Q139C(c.415C>T)	severe(20-60mmol/L)	ApoA5*3 (with S19W) or the APOA5*2 haplotype	late onset of hyperchylomicronemia	[59]
Q97X(c.289C>T)	mild to extreme	promoter of ApoC3 gene (-**482C/C)**	hyperchylomicronemia, xanthomas, , might be associated with pancreatitis	[60]
E255G(c.764A>G)	extreme(75mmol/L)	S19W ,homozygous for LPL W86G	pregnancy associated hypertriglyceridemia	[63]
G271C(c.811G>T)	severe (20 mmol/L)	A315V , -1131C, S19W	pancreatitis	[63]
H321L(c.962A>T)	extreme(63mmol/L)	A315V, S19W, LPL-P207L	pancreatitis, DM2	[63]
N66S(c.197A>G)	severe			[65]
G185C(c.553G>T)	severe	S19W, -3A>G	common in Asian population recently identified in Caucasion polputation	[65.66]
Q305X(c.937C>T)	severe			[65]
A315V(c.944C>T)	mild to extreme	S19W, severe HTG patient carry the N291S LPL SNP	Type III hyperlipidemia, DM2	[67]
L242P(c.725T>C)	severe (35mmol/L)	various known haplotypes	might be associated with metabolic syndrome	[71]
Q145R(c.434A>G)	severe (over10mmol/L)			[67]
E255K(c.763G>A)	severe (over10mmol/L)			[67]
E52K(c.154G>A)	moderate (below10mmol/L)			[67]
Q252H(c.756G>C)	severe (10mmol/L)	S19W		[67]
R301P(c.902G>C)	extreme (76 mmol/L)	L314 mutation, S19W		[67]
Q95X(c.283C>T)	moderate (below10mmol/L)			[67]
Q295X(c.883C>T)	moderate (9mmol/L))	not known	Type III Hyperlipidemia	[67]
G165D(c.494G>A)	severe(10mmol/L)			[67]

A very recent resequencing study was performed in 2011 by Evans et al [67] to determine the frequency of rare variant of the *ApoA5* gene in patient with different types of HTG was done in. The study involved 291 patients with HTG from which 98 had TG levels above 875mg/dl, 111 patients with ApoE2/2 genotype from whom 100 had Type III hyperlipidemia, and 108 healthy controls. From the 98 patients with severe HTG (875mg/dl+) only 23 had neither variants in their *ApoA5* or *LPL* gene. Evans et al. found several novel point mutations in patients with severe HTG from which according to Polyphen analysis p.Q145R, p.E255K was thought to be benign, p.Q252H possibly damaging, p.R301P, p.L314R (same patient) probably damaging. Some of the patient had a deletion creating a frameshift from the severe HTH group: c427delC and c722delC and one proband with an insertion frameshift c.999-28bpins was identified.

In the moderate HTG group (< 875mg/dl>95th percentile) the novel p.E52K variant is thought to be benign, the p.G165D is probably damaging, and the novel p.Q95X nonsense mutation most likely result in a premature truncation thus creating LPL-ApoA5 interaction defect. They also found one deletion in the moderate group: c978-979delAG and inframe deletion: c922-924delGAG. From the Type III hyperlipidemic patient one carried a novel nonsense mutation: p.Q295X. This study also showed that ApoA5 rare mutations are significantly more prevalent in severe HTGH patient compared to healthy controls. Table 2 summarizes the known point mutations, and known genetic data about them. Clinical relevancy is also indicated in known cases.

The first intronic mutation causing HTG and reduced LPL activity was described by Olivia et al. in an earlier phase of the ApoA5 research [68]. Screening 32 patients with HTG, a 51 year old male and his father were found to be carrying a mutation at the c161+3- position in heterozygous form. In vitro analysis of the g.IVS3+3G>C mutation leads to an exon splice-site skipping, resulting in the deletion of the third exon, thus creating a frame shift, which introduces premature termination. Paradoxically, the patient's ApoA5 level was in a normal range.

Table 3. Splicing Mutations of Apolipoprotein A5

Splicing Mutation	TG	Association	Clinical relevance	Ref
IVS2+1G>A(c.49+1G>A)	severe (20mmol/L)	ApoA5*2	Pancreatitis	[70]
IVS3+3G>C(c.161+3G>)	severe (19.9mmol/L)	T361T;-1131T/C c.56C/C,homozygous for the rare allele in the promoter of ApoC3(−482 T/T)		[68]
IVS3+5G>C			Pregnancy associated hypertriglyceridemia	[69]
IVS3-43G>A				[2]

The second intronic mutation was found in ApoA5 deficient patient, whose HTG was estrogen induced, and the underlying cause for this phenotype was a g.IVS3+5G>C mutation [69]. The most novel mutation involving splicing was discovered in a Japanese patient with chylomycronemia [70]. The patient was a 54 year-old male, diagnosed with HTG at the age of 35. His TG level was over a 1000 mg/dl he was on fibrate therapy. The underlying cause was a mutation in the c.49+1 position. The g.IVS2+1G>A genotype, according to splice site analysis completely abolishes the function of the donor splice site in intron 2. The patient was also carrying the well known TG level lifter ApoA5*2 haplotype. Mutations affecting splicing are summarized in Table 3.

Table 4. Deletion/Insertion mutations of Apolipoprotein A5

Deletion Frameshift	TG	Reference
c427delC	severe (over10mmol/L) moderate	[67]
	below(10mmol/L)	
c722delC	severe (over10mmol/L)	[67]
c978-979delAG	severe (875-100 mg /dl)	[67]
Insertion Frameshift	TG	Reference
c999-28bpins	severe (over10mmol/L)	[67]

There are also several known deleterious and insertion mutations of ApoA5. All of them were described by Evans et al [67]. These mutations are associated with highly elevated TG levels. They are summarized in Table 4.

Conclusion

In the past decade significant progress has been achieved in the ApoA 5 research, it as it plays an effective phisiological regulatory role in triglyceride metabolism at a moderate rage of circulating plasma ApoA5 concentration. Associated with this key role of the ApoA5, the common naturally occurring haplotype tagging variants (T-1131C, T1259C, C56G, and IVS3+G476A) and ApoA5 haplotypes determined by them, are associated with elevated plasma triglyceride concentrations, these variants and haplotype combinations have been shown to confer risk or protection for development of cardiovascular disease, stroke and metabolic syndrome. It also became clear, that there are also some less frequent genetic variants, which in combination with the common allelic variants of the gene can define haplotypes that are associated with higher triglyceride levels. The test of these variants can now be found in the palette of the direct-to-consumer services; interpretation of these results requires precaution. Clinically importantly, there are rare mutations of the *ApoA5* gene which are associated with specific complex rare-disease phenotype that can include even extremely high triglyceride levels with multiple organ pathology; the spectrum of the likely will further increase.

Acknowledgment

The experimental part of this review was supported by the grant of OTKA 73430.

References

[1] van der Vliet HN; Sammels MG; Leegwater AC; Levels JH; Reitsma PH; Boers W; Chamuleau RA. Apolipoprotein A-V: a novel apolipoprotein associated with an early phase of liver regeneration. *J. Biol. Chem.,* 2001, 276, 44512-44520.

[2] Pennacchio LA; Olivier M; Hubacek JA; Cohen JC; Cox DR; Fruchart JC; Krauss RM; Rubin EM. An apolipoprotein influencing triglycerides in humans and mice revealed by comparative sequencing. *Science,* 2001, 294, 169-173.

[3] Weinberg RB; Cook VR; Beckstead JA; Martin DD; Gallagher JW; Shelness GS; Ryan RO. Structure and interfacial properties of human apolipoprotein A-V. *J. Biol. Chem.,* 2003, 278, 34438-34444.

[4] Kujiraoka T; Oka T; Ishihara M; Egashira T; Fujioka T; Saito E; Saito S; Miller NE; Hattori H. A sandwich enzyme-linked immunosorbent assay for human serum paraoxonase concentration. *J. Lipid. Res.,* 2000, 41, 1358-1363.

[5] O'Brien PJ; Alborn WE; Sloan JH; Ulmer M; Boodhoo A; Knierman MD; Schultze AE; Konrad RJ. The novel apolipoprotein A5 is present in human serum, is associated with VLDL, HDL, and chylomicrons, and circulates at very low concentrations compared with other apolipoproteins. *Clin. Chem.,* 2005, 51, 351-359.

[6] Merkel M and Heeren J. Give me A5 for lipoprotein hydrolysis! *J. Clin. Invest.,* 2005, 115, 2694-2696.

[7] Beckstead JA; Oda MN; Martin DD; Forte TM; Bielicki JK; Berger T; Luty R; Kay CM; Ryan RO. Structure-function studies of human apolipoprotein A-V: a regulator of plasma lipid homeostasis. *Biochemistry,* 2003, 42, 9416-9423.

[8] Nilsson SK; Heeren J; Olivecrona G; Merkel M. Apolipoprotein A-V; a potent triglyceride reducer. *Atherosclerosis,* 2011, 219, 15-21.

[9] Wong-Mauldin K; Raussens V; Forte TM; Ryan RO. Apolipoprotein A-V N-terminal domain lipid interaction properties in vitro explain the hypertriglyceridemic phenotype associated with natural truncation mutants. *J. Biol. Chem.,* 2009, 284, 33369-33376.

[10] Wong K; Beckstead JA; Lee D; Weers PM; Guigard E; Kay CM; Ryan RO. The N-terminus of apolipoprotein A-V adopts a helix bundle molecular architecture. *Biochemistry,* 2008, 47, 8768-8774.

[11] Sun G; Bi N; Li G; Zhu X; Zeng W; Wu G; Xue H; Chen B. Identification of lipid binding and lipoprotein lipase activation domains of human apoAV. *Chem. Phys. Lipids,* 2006, 143, 22-28.

[12] Gin P; Beigneux AP; Davies B; Young MF; Ryan RO; Bensadoun A; Fong LG; Young SG. Normal binding of lipoprotein lipase, chylomicrons, and apo-AV to GPIHBP1 containing a G56R amino acid substitution. *Biochim. Biophys. Acta,* 2007, 1771, 1464-1468.

[13] Gin P; Yin L; Davies BS; Weinstein MM; Ryan RO; Bensadoun A; Fong LG; Young SG; Beigneux AP. The acidic domain of GPIHBP1 is important for the binding of lipoprotein lipase and chylomicrons. *J. Biol. Chem.,* 2008, 283, 29554-29562.

[14] Sharma V; Ryan RO; Forte TM. Apolipoprotein A-V dependent modulation of plasma triacylglycerol: A puzzlement. *Biochim. Biophys. Acta,* 2012, 1821, 795-799.

[15] Alborn WE; Johnson MG; Prince MJ; Konrad RJ. Definitive N-terminal protein sequence and further characterization of the novel apolipoprotein A5 in human serum. *Clin. Chem.,* 2006, 52, 514-517.

[16] Lookene A; Nielsen MS; Gliemann J; Olivecrona G. Contribution of the carboxy-terminal domain of lipoprotein lipase to interaction with heparin and lipoproteins. *Biochem. Biophys. Res. Commun.,* 2000, 271, 15-21.

[17] Nilsson SK; Lookene A; Beckstead JA; Gliemann J; Ryan RO; Olivecrona G. Apolipoprotein A-V interaction with members of the low density lipoprotein receptor gene family. *Biochemistry,* 2007, 46, 3896-3904.

[18] Lookene A; Beckstead JA; Nilsson S; Olivecrona G; Ryan RO. Apolipoprotein A-V-heparin interactions: implications for plasma lipoprotein metabolism. *J. Biol. Chem.,* 2005, 280, 25383-25387.

[19] Helleboid-Chapman A; Nowak M; Helleboid S; Moitrot E; Rommens C; Dehondt H; Heliot L; Drobecq H; Fruchart-Najib J; Fruchart JC. Apolipoprotein A-V modulates insulin secretion in pancreatic beta-cells through its interaction with midkine. *Cell Physiol. Biochem.,* 2009, 24, 451-460.

[20] Grosskopf I; Baroukh N; Lee SJ; Kamari Y; Harats D; Rubin EM; Pennacchio LA; Cooper AD. Apolipoprotein A-V deficiency results in marked hypertriglyceridemia attributable to decreased lipolysis of triglyceride-rich lipoproteins and removal of their remnants. *Arterioscler. Thromb. Vasc. Biol.,* 2005, 25, 2573-2579.

[21] Aalto-Setala K; Fisher EA; Chen X; Chajek-Shaul T; Hayek T; Zechner R; Walsh A; Ramakrishnan R; Ginsberg HN; Breslow JL. Mechanism of hypertriglyceridemia in human apolipoprotein (apo) CIII transgenic mice. Diminished very low density lipoprotein fractional catabolic rate associated with increased apo CIII and reduced apo E on the particles. *J. Clin. Invest.,* 1992, 90, 1889-1900.

[22] Baroukh N; Bauge E; Akiyama J; Chang J; Afzal V; Fruchart JC; Rubin EM; Fruchart-Najib J; Pennacchio LA. Analysis of apolipoprotein A5, c3, and plasma triglyceride concentrations in genetically engineered mice. *Arterioscler. Thromb. Vasc. Biol.,* 2004, 24, 1297-1302.

[23] Schaap FG; Nierman MC; Berbee JF; Hattori H; Talmud PJ; Vaessen SF; Rensen PC; Chamuleau RA; Kuivenhoven JA; Groen AK. Evidence for a complex relationship between apoA-V and apoC-III in patients with severe hypertriglyceridemia. *J. Lipid. Res.,* 2006, 47, 2333-2339.

[24] Merkel M; Loeffler B; Kluger M; Fabig N; Geppert G; Pennacchio LA; Laatsch A; Heeren J. Apolipoprotein AV accelerates plasma hydrolysis of triglyceride-rich lipoproteins by interaction with proteoglycan-bound lipoprotein lipase. *J. Biol. Chem.,* 2005, 280, 21553-21560.

[25] Kluger M; Heeren J; Merkel M. Apoprotein A-V: An important regulator of triglyceride metabolism. *J. Inherit. Metab. Dis.,* 2008.

[26] van Dijk KW; Rensen PC; Voshol PJ; Havekes LM. The role and mode of action of apolipoproteins CIII and AV: synergistic actors in triglyceride metabolism? *Curr. Opin. Lipidol.,* 2004, 15, 239-246.

[27] Zhang Z; Peng B; Gong RR; Gao LB; Du J; Fang DZ; Song YY; Li YH; Ou GJ. Apolipoprotein A5 polymorphisms and risk of coronary artery disease: a meta-analysis. *Biosci. Trends,* 2011, 5, 165-172.

[28] Pennacchio LA; Olivier M; Hubacek JA; Krauss RM; Rubin EM; Cohen JC. Two independent apolipoprotein A5 haplotypes influence human plasma triglyceride levels. *Hum. Mol. Genet.,* 2002, 11, 3031-3038.
[29] Cullen P. Evidence that triglycerides are an independent coronary heart disease risk factor. *Am. J. Cardiol.,* 2000, 86, 943-949.
[30] Talmud PJ; Hawe E; Miller GJ; Humphries SE. Nonfasting apolipoprotein B and triglyceride levels as a useful predictor of coronary heart disease risk in middle-aged UK men. *Arterioscler. Thromb. Vasc. Biol.,* 2002, 22, 1918-1923.
[31] Chandak GR; Ward KJ; Yajnik CS; Pandit AN; Bavdekar A; Joglekar CV; Fall CH; Mohankrishna P; Wilkin TJ; Metcalf BS; Weedon MN; Frayling TM; Hattersley AT. Triglyceride associated polymorphisms of the APOA5 gene have very different allele frequencies in Pune, India compared to Europeans. *BMC Med. Genet.,* 2006, 7, 76.
[32] Maasz A; Kisfali P; Horvatovich K; Mohas M; Marko L; Csongei V; Farago B; Jaromi L; Magyari L; Safrany E; Sipeky C; Wittmann I; Melegh B. Apolipoprotein A5 T-1131C variant confers risk for metabolic syndrome. *Pathol. Oncol. Res.,* 2007, 13, 243-247.
[33] Kisfali P; Mohas M; Maasz A; Polgar N; Hadarits F; Marko L; Brasnyo P; Horvatovich K; Oroszlan T; Bagosi Z; Bujtor Z; Gasztonyi B; Rinfel J; Wittmann I; Melegh B. Haplotype analysis of the apolipoprotein A5 gene in patients with the metabolic syndrome. *Nutr. Metab. Cardiovasc. Dis.,* 2010, 20, 505-511.
[34] Niculescu LS; Fruchart-Najib J; Fruchart JC; Sima A. Apolipoprotein A-V gene polymorphisms in subjects with metabolic syndrome. *Clin. Chem. Lab. Med.,* 2007, 45, 1133-1139.
[35] Dallinga-Thie GM; van TA; Hattori H; van Vark-van der Zee LC; Jansen H; Sijbrands EJ. Plasma apolipoprotein A5 and triglycerides in type 2 diabetes. *Diabetologia,* 2006, 49, 1505-1511.
[36] Henneman P; Schaap FG; Havekes LM; Rensen PC; Frants RR; van TA; Hattori H; Smelt AH; van Dijk KW. Plasma apoAV levels are markedly elevated in severe hypertriglyceridemia and positively correlated with the APOA5 S19W polymorphism. *Atherosclerosis,* 2007, 193, 129-134.
[37] Talmud PJ; Cooper JA; Hattori H; Miller IP; Miller GJ; Humphries SE. The apolipoprotein A-V genotype and plasma apolipoprotein A-V and triglyceride levels: prospective risk of type 2 diabetes. Results from the Northwick Park Heart Study II. *Diabetologia,* 2006, 49, 2337-2340.
[38] Vaessen SF; Schaap FG; Kuivenhoven JA; Groen AK; Hutten BA; Boekholdt SM; Hattori H; Sandhu MS; Bingham SA; Luben R; Palmen JA; Wareham NJ; Humphries SE; Kastelein JJ; Talmud PJ; Khaw KT. Apolipoprotein A-V, triglycerides and risk of coronary artery disease: the prospective Epic-Norfolk Population Study. *J. Lipid. Res.,* 2006, 47, 2064-2070.
[39] Tai ES and Ordovas JM. Clinical significance of apolipoprotein A5. *Curr. Opin. Lipidol.,* 2008, 19, 349-354.
[40] Sarwar N; Sandhu MS; Ricketts SL; Butterworth AS; Di AE; Boekholdt SM; Ouwehand W; Watkins H; Samani NJ; Saleheen D; Lawlor D; Reilly MP; Hingorani AD; Talmud PJ; Danesh J. Triglyceride-mediated pathways and coronary disease: collaborative analysis of 101 studies. *Lancet,* 2010, 375, 1634-1639.

[41] Yu Y; Xue L; Zhao CY. [Study on polymorphism in the apolipoprotein A5 gene in patients with premature coronary heart disease]. *Beijing Da Xue Xue Bao,* 2007, 39, 576-580.

[42] Havasi V; Szolnoki Z; Talian G; Bene J; Komlosi K; Maasz A; Somogyvari F; Kondacs A; Szabo M; Fodor L; Bodor A; Melegh B. Apolipoprotein A5 gene promoter region T-1131C polymorphism associates with elevated circulating triglyceride levels and confers susceptibility for development of ischemic stroke. *J. Mol. Neurosci.,* 2006, 29, 177-183.

[43] Arnedo M; Taffe P; Sahli R; Furrer H; Hirschel B; Elzi L; Weber R; Vernazza P; Bernasconi E; Darioli R; Bergmann S; Beckmann JS; Telenti A; Tarr PE. Contribution of 20 single nucleotide polymorphisms of 13 genes to dyslipidemia associated with antiretroviral therapy. *Pharmacogenet. Genomics,* 2007, 17,755-764.

[44] Horinek A; Vrablik M; Ceska R; Adamkova V; Poledne R; Hubacek JA. T-1131-->C polymorphism within the apolipoprotein AV gene in hypertriglyceridemic individuals. *Atherosclerosis,* 003,167, 369-370.

[45] Hubacek JA; Adamkova V; Vrablik M; Kadlecova M; Zicha J; Kunes J; Pitha J; Suchanek P; Poledne R. Apolipoprotein A5 in health and disease. *Physiol. Res.,* 2009,58 Suppl 2,S101-S109.

[46] Hubacek JA. Apolipoprotein A5 and triglyceridemia. Focus on the effects of the common variants. *Clin. Chem. Lab. Med.,* 2005, 43, 897-902.

[47] Hubacek JA; Skodova Z; Adamkova V; Lanska V; Poledne R. The influence of APOAV polymorphisms (T-1131>C and S19>W) on plasma triglyceride levels and risk of myocardial infarction. *Clin. Genet.,* 2004, 65, 126-130.

[48] Yang Y; Ruiz-Narvaez E; Niu T; Xu X; Campos H. Genetic variants of the lipoprotein lipase gene and myocardial infarction in the Central Valley of Costa Rica. *J. Lipid. Res.,* 2004, 45, 2106-2109.

[49] Wright WT; Young IS; Nicholls DP; Patterson C; Lyttle K; Graham CA. SNPs at the APOA5 gene account for the strong association with hypertriglyceridaemia at the APOA5/A4/C3/A1 locus on chromosome 11q23 in the Northern Irish population. *Atherosclerosis,* 2006, 185, 353-360.

[50] Maasz A; Kisfali P; Jaromi L; Horvatovich K; Szolnoki Z; Csongei V; Safrany E; Sipeky C; Hadarits F; Melegh B. Apolipoprotein A5 gene IVS3+G476A allelic variant confers susceptibility for development of ischemic stroke. *Circ. J.,* 2008, 72, 1065-1070.

[51] Kisfali P; Mohas M; Maasz A; Hadarits F; Marko L; Horvatovich K; Oroszlan T; Bagosi Z; Bujtor Z; Gasztonyi B; Wittmann I; Melegh B. Apolipoprotein A5 IVS3+476A allelic variant associates with increased trigliceride levels and confers risk for development of metabolic syndrome in Hungarians. *Circ. J.,* 2008, 72, 40-43.

[52] Lai CQ; Tai ES; Tan CE; Cutter J; Chew SK; Zhu YP; Adiconis X; Ordovas JM. The APOA5 locus is a strong determinant of plasma triglyceride concentrations across ethnic groups in Singapore. *J. Lipid. Res.,* 2003, 44, 2365-2373.

[53] Maasz A; Kisfali P; Szolnoki Z; Hadarits F; Melegh B. Apolipoprotein A5 gene C56G variant confers risk for the development of large-vessel associated ischemic stroke. *J. Neurol.,* 2008, 255, 649-654.

[54] Horvatovich K; Bokor S; Barath A; Maasz A; Kisfali P; Jaromi L; Polgar N; Toth D; Repasy J; Endreffy E; Molnar D; Melegh B. Haplotype analysis of the apolipoprotein A5 gene in obese pediatric patients. *Int. J. Pediatr. Obes.*, 2011,6,e318-e325.

[55] Brunzell JD. *Familial Lipoprotein Lipase Deficiency*. 1993.

[56] Durrington P. Dyslipidaemia. *Lancet,* 2003, 362, 717-731.

[57] Priore OC; Pisciotta L; Li VG; Sambataro MP; Cantafora A; Bellocchio A; Catapano A; Tarugi P; Bertolini S; Calandra S. Inherited apolipoprotein A-V deficiency in severe hypertriglyceridemia. *Arterioscler. Thromb. Vasc. Biol.*, 2005, 25, 411-417.

[58] Talmud PJ; Hawe E; Martin S; Olivier M; Miller GJ; Rubin EM; Pennacchio LA; Humphries SE. Relative contribution of variation within the APOC3/A4/A5 gene cluster in determining plasma triglycerides. *Hum. Mol. Genet.,* 2002, 11, 3039-3046.

[59] Marcais C; Verges B; Charriere S; Pruneta V; Merlin M; Billon S; Perrot L; Drai J; Sassolas A; Pennacchio LA; Fruchart-Najib J; Fruchart JC; Durlach V; Moulin P. Apoa5 Q139X truncation predisposes to late-onset hyperchylomicronemia due to lipoprotein lipase impairment. *J. Clin. Invest.,* 2005, 115, 2862-2869.

[60] Priore OC; Carubbi F; Schaap FG; Bertolini S; Calandra S. Hypertriglyceridaemia and low plasma HDL in a patient with apolipoprotein A-V deficiency due to a novel mutation in the APOA5 gene. *J. Intern. Med.,* 2008, 263, 450-458.

[61] Wang CS; McConathy WJ; Kloer HU; Alaupovic P. Modulation of lipoprotein lipase activity by apolipoproteins. Effect of apolipoprotein C-III. *J. Clin. Invest.,* 1985, 75, 384-390.

[62] Qu S; Perdomo G; Su D; D'Souza FM; Shachter NS; Dong HH. Effects of apoA-V on HDL and VLDL metabolism in APOC3 transgenic mice. *J. Lipid. Res.,* 2007, 48, 1476-1487.

[63] Dorfmeister B; Zeng WW; Dichlberger A; Nilsson SK; Schaap FG; Hubacek JA; Merkel M; Cooper JA; Lookene A; Putt W; Whittall R; Lee PJ; Lins L; Delsaux N; Nierman M; Kuivenhoven JA; Kastelein JJ; Vrablik M; Olivecrona G; Schneider WJ; Heeren J; Humphries SE; Talmud PJ. Effects of six APOA5 variants, identified in patients with severe hypertriglyceridemia, on in vitro lipoprotein lipase activity and receptor binding. *Arterioscler. Thromb. Vasc. Biol.,* 2008,28, 1866-1871.

[64] Mailly F; Palmen J; Muller DP; Gibbs T; Lloyd J; Brunzell J; Durrington P; Mitropoulos K; Betteridge J; Watts G; Lithell H; Angelico F; Humphries SE; Talmud PJ. Familial lipoprotein lipase (LPL) deficiency: a catalogue of LPL gene mutations identified in 20 patients from the UK, Sweden, and Italy. *Hum. Mutat.,* 1997, 10, 465-473.

[65] Johansen CT; Wang J; Lanktree MB; Cao H; McIntyre AD; Ban MR; Martins RA; Kennedy BA; Hassell RG; Visser ME; Schwartz SM; Voight BF; Elosua R; Salomaa V; O'Donnell CJ; Dallinga-Thie GM; Anand SS; Yusuf S; Huff MW; Kathiresan S; Hegele RA. Excess of rare variants in genes identified by genome-wide association study of hypertriglyceridemia. *Nat. Genet.,* 2010, 42,684-687.

[66] Kao JT; Wen HC; Chien KL; Hsu HC; Lin SW. A novel genetic variant in the apolipoprotein A5 gene is associated with hypertriglyceridemia. *Hum. Mol. Genet.,* 2003, 12, 2533-2539.

[67] Evans D; Aberle J; Beil FU. Resequencing the Apolipoprotein A5 (APOA5) gene in patients with various forms of hypertriglyceridemia. *Atherosclerosis,* 2011, 219, 715-720.

[68] Priore OC; Tarugi P; Calandra S; Pisciotta L; Bellocchio A; Bertolini S; Guardamagna O; Schaap FG. A novel sequence variant in APOA5 gene found in patients with severe hypertriglyceridemia. *Atherosclerosis,* 2006, 188, 215-217.

[69] Henneman P; Schaap FG; Rensen PC; van Dijk KW; Smelt AH. Estrogen induced hypertriglyceridemia in an apolipoprotein AV deficient patient. *J. Intern. Med.,* 2008, 263, 107-108.

[70] Okubo M; Ishihara M; Iwasaki T; Ebara T; Aoyama Y; Murase T; Hattori H. A novel APOA5 splicing mutation IVS2+1g>a in a Japanese chylomicronemia patient. *Atherosclerosis,* 2009, 207, 24-25.

[71] Charriere S; Cugnet C; Guitard M; Bernard S; Groisne L; Charcosset M; Pruneta-Deloche V; Merlin M; Billon S; Delay M; Sassolas A; Moulin P; Marcais C. Modulation of phenotypic expression of APOA5 Q97X and L242P mutations. *Atherosclerosis,* 2009, 207, 150-156.

In: Apolipoproteins
Editors: A. D. Sidorov and M. Y. Nikitin
ISBN: 978-1-62257-484-1

Chapter V

Mechanism of Antiinflammatory Action of the High Density Lipoproteins and Apolipoprotein A-I

L. Polyakov, D. Sumenkova and L. Panin
Institute of Biochemistry,
Siberian Division of the Russian Academy of Medical Science, Novosibirsk, Russia

Abstract

It is known that lipoproteins and lipopolysaccharide binding protein bind lipopolysaccharide in blood plasma and play important role in the mechanism of anti-inflammatory protection. The aim of the present study was to investigate the role of high-density lipoproteins and apolipoprotein A-I in binding, transport and neutralization of bacterial lipopolysaccharide. We used the high-density lipoproteins (HDL), apolipoprotein A-I (apoA-I), rat hepatocytes, tumor-associated macrophages (TAMs), and lipopolysaccharide (LPS) from Escherichia coli. To study interactions of LPS and HDL we used tryptophan fluorescence quenching and electrophoretic mobilities in agarose gel. Our results suggest a physical interaction of HDL with LPS. ApoA-I, the main protein component of HDL, plays a crucial role in LPS binding to HDL. Pathological effect of LPS is mediated by proinflammatory cytokines secreted by macrophages. The increased secretion of some cytokines is harmful for neighboring cells. For example, the ability of IL-1β to increase metastatic potential of a tumor is well known. It is considered that interaction of HDL with LPS prevent the activation of macrophages. We found that the treatment of TAMs culture with LPS-HDL complexes decreased an intracellular IL-1β concentration in TAMs. The effect of HDL may be caused by participation of apoA-I in regulation of expression of genes of proinflammatory cytokines in macrophages or with endocytosis of LPS with HDL through macrophages HDL-receptors, without participation Toll-like receptor and activation of cytokine genes. Using the fluorescent microscopy and spectrofluorimetry we found the ability of apoA-I to carry fluorescein isothiocyanate labeled LPS into rat hepatocytes. It is known, that LPS does not interact directly with hepatocytes. We suppose that complex LPS with apoA-I interacts with a HDL-receptor and gets into cells by endocytosis and then can be exposed to metabolic degradation in hepatocytes. Our date indicates that hepatocytes take place in LPS clearance as a complex with HDL bypassing macrophages. Neutralization of LPS by HDL can be considered as alternative and safe way, allowing to prevent an activation of macrophages and decreases the inflammatory response. The results of the present study demonstrate that HDL and apoA-I may play an important role in LPS binding and prevent acute inflammatory response and development of metabolic diseases.

Introduction

Numerous studies have demonstrated that all lipoprotein classes bind lipopolysaccharide (LPS, endotoxin) from the outer surface membrane of gram-negative bacteria and as well as lipopolysaccharide binding protein (LBP) transfer LPS in blood [1 – 3]. In normal lipidemic animals, 63% of LPS in plasma is associated with lipoproteins. In contrast, in hypolipidemic animals, about 17% LPS is associated with lipoproteins [4]. It was found that lipoproteins bound LPS in direct proportion to their plasma cholesterol concentration [5].

This binding to lipoproteins inhibits the ability of LPS to activate macrophages. It is know that after entering the bloodstream, LPS will bind to LBP, which helps in transferring LPS to co-receptor CD14 on cells of the monocyte/macrophage lineage, leading to the formation of receptor clusters of Toll-like receptor 4 (TLR4), CD14, and other adaptors, resulting in the activation of the nuclear factor NF-kB pathway and production of a cascade of proinflammatory cytokines, such as TNF-α, IL-1β, and IL-6, which mediate the cellular inflammatory response to Gram-negative infection [6, 7]. Systemic release of these mediators during bacteremia or overwhelming Gram-negative infection can lead to septic shock and death.

Several studies suggest that mainly high density lipoprotein (HDL) binds LPS and neutralizes its toxicity. Moreover, apolipoprotein A-I (apoA-I) is the major contributor for HDL anti-endotoxin function, and lipoprotein-free plasma fraction enhances the effect of apoA-I [8]. Additionally, apoA-I is a key component in the association of LBP with HDL and may play an important role in the biologic activity of LPS/LBP complexes [9].

Numerous studies have demonstrated that HDL and apoA-I play an important role in host defense against endotoxemia and infection. Humans with low HDL levels have a more robust inflammatory response to LPS administration [10]. The administration of reconstituted HDL to humans blunts the deleterious effects of LPS administration [11]. Transgenic mice overexpressing apoA-I have elevations in serum HDL levels and are protected from severe bacterial infection and LPS-induced death [12]. Similarly, several studies have shown that infusion of HDL or apoA-I mimetic peptides into animals with experimental sepsis decreases TNF production and improves survival [13, 14]. Other studies demonstrate that apoAI mimetic peptide L-4F reduces the expression of inflammatory markers induced by LPS. The inhibitory effect of L-4F was associated with reduced binding of LPS to its plasma carrier molecule (LBP), and decreased binding of LPS to cells. Furthermore, the studies suggest a physical interaction between LPS and apoA-I mimetic peptide [15]. Our laboratory has previously shown that HDL3 and apoA-I decrease the LPS-induced production of reactive oxygen intermediates in Kupffer cells isolated from livers of zymosan-treated rats more than low density lipoproteins [16]. Furthermore, HDL3 prevents LPS-induced liver injury in zymosan-pretreated rats [17].

ApoA-I alone can neutralize LPS and this interaction can be altered by changing the structure of apoA-I [18]. However, several studies show that phospholipid content of lipoproteins also plays a key role [19]. For example, the studies of Hara et al. demonstrate that the phospholipid content of HDL from endothelial lipase knockout mice is increased and that the increased protection from LPS-induced toxicity is proportional to the increase in phospholipids rather than an increase in HDL protein [20]. Thus, both apolipoproteins and phospholipids can play important roles in the ability of HDL to neutralize LPS.

The mechanisms of protection against endotoxin by HDL and apoA-I remain poorly understood. It is clear that interaction of HDL with LPS prevents the activation of macrophages and a strong cytokine response to LPS. Probably, LPS complexed with HDL disappears more slowly from the circulation. Undoubtedly that the liver is the main organ that clears circulating LPS. However, controversy remains regarding the relative roles of Kupffer cells and hepatocytes in the uptake and clearance of free LPS and lipoprotein-bound LPS. The studies of Treon et al. suggested that LPS are preferentially taken up by Kupffer cells and deacylated, which then allows for more rapid internalization within hepatocytes [21]. Other studies using gadolinium chloride to deplete Kupffer cells have determined that hepatocytes also play a major role in LPS clearance [22], and deacylation of LPS also takes place in hepatocytes [23]. Hepatic uptake mechanisms are actively studied now. Some results suggested the presence of a lectin-like receptor for the LPS on the plasma membrane of rat hepatocytes [24]. It was found the uptake not to be receptor-mediated [25]. Other studies indicate that hepatocytes express the cell surface components of the LPS receptor/signaling complex (CD14/TLR4/MD2) and that signaling activated by LPS through this receptor complex on hepatocytes leads to the activation of MAPK signaling proteins, translocation of NFκB to the nucleus, and also production and release of acute phase proteins such as soluble CD14 and LPS-binding protein [26, 27]. Finally, this complex plays a role in the binding and initiation of uptake of LPS into cells [28]. The new studies of Shao B. et al. suggest that only Kupffer cells play important role in clearing and catabolizing both free LPS and HDL-bound LPS [29].

Thus, the mechanisms involved in the internalization of LPS remain uncertain and controversial. From the point of our view the mechanisms of protection against endotoxin by HDL and apoA-I can be associated with existence of an alternative way for endotoxin metabolic degradation via the HDL-receptor pathways, in particular scavenger receptors. It is shown that SR-BI is a critical protective modulator of sepsis in mice. SR-BI exerts its protective function through its role in modulating inflammatory response in macrophages and facilitating LPS recruitment and clearance [30].

In this study we have demonstrated that lipoproteins of different classes and apoA-I bind bacterial and yeast polysaccharides and decrease IL-1β production by tumor-associated macrophages (TAMs) and prevent the activation of polysaccharide-treated TAMs. We have also shown that apoA-I can be the LPS carrier into isolated hepatocytes of rat.

Materials and Methods

Isolation of lipoproteins from blood serum. Lipoproteins were isolated from rat and human blood serum by isodensity ultracentrifugation in KBr solutions in the presence of 3 mM EDTA-Na_2 using an Optima L-90K (Beckman Coulter, Austria) centrifuge with a 70.1

Ti rotor [31]. Three main lipoprotein fractions were obtained: very low density lipoproteins (VLDL, 0.94 < d < 1.006 g/ml), low density lipoproteins (LDL, 1.006 < d < 1.063 g/ml), and high density lipoproteins (HDL, 1.063 < d < 1.21 g/ml). The obtained lipoproteins were dialyzed for 24 h at 4°C against 0.05 M potassium-phosphate buffer, pH 7.4, containing 0.15 M NaCl and 0.3 mM EDTA-Na_2, then sterilized by filtering through Millipore filters (USA, 22 μm pore diameter).

Isolation of apolipoprotein A-I. HDL was delipidated in a chilled chloroform-methanol mixture (1:1), 20 ml of the mixture per 1 ml of lipoproteins, which was followed by multiple washing in ether [32]. To obtain apolipoprotein A-I, total HDL proteins in solution of 3% Ds-Na and 0.1% mercaptoethanol were deposited on a column (1.6 x 100 cm) of Sepharose 6B-CL (Pharmacia, Sweden) and eluted with 5 mM Tris buffer, pH 8.6, containing 6 M urea, 0.01% sodium azide and 1 mM phenylmethanesulfonyl fluoride (PMSF). The flow rate was 10 ml/h, and a recorder was operated at 9 mm/h. The elution profile was recorded on UV detector 2151 LKB (Sweden) at wavelength 280 nm. Purity of apoA-I was checked by electrophoresis in 12.5% SDS-PAGE. Protein strips were visualized by 0.1% Coomassie G-250 in a mixture of methanol and 10% acetic acid (1:1). A set of low-molecular weight protein standards (phosphorylase, 94 kDa; albumin, 67 kDa; ovalbumin, 43 kDa; carboanhydrase, 30 kDa; and lactalbumin, 14.4 kDa) were used as markers.

HDL and apoA-I were desalted by gel filtration on a 20 x 0.8 cm column of Sephadex G-25 (Pharmacia, Sweden); eluent: 5 mM Tris-HCl buffer, pH 7.4, ontaining 0.15 M NaCl; the elution rate 30 ml/h, recorder operated at 9 cm/h). The elution profile was recorded on a UV detector at wavelength 280 nm.

Agarose electrophoresis. The electrophoretic mobilities of different lipoproteins and apolipoprotein A-I were determined by electrophoresis on preformed 1% agarose gel. Samples in Tris/NaCl, pH 8 were applied to gel wells and allowed to penetrate into the gel for 5 min before the electric field was applied. Power supply was used to apply a voltage of 100 volts across a gel distance of 5.5 cm. Electrophoresis was continued for 30 min at 25°C in the kit barbital buffer (pH 8.6, 0.05 ionic strength). After electrophoresis, the gels were fixed in a solution of ethanol-acetic acid-water 60:10:30 (v/v/v), oven dried (80°C for 1 h) and then stained (5 min) with a 0.15% Coomassie Blue R250 solution. Gels were destained in a solution of methanol-acetic acid-water 35:25:40 (v/v/v) for about 10 min.

Isolation of hepatocytes. The procedure for isolation of hepatocytes included the following steps: 1 – in situ perfusion of the liver by Ca^{2+}-free Hanks solution to remove blood from the organ; 2 – recirculating perfusion of the liver in vitro by a collagenase solution for proteolytic digestion of connective tissue; 3 – mechanical disaggregation of the tissue; 4 – differential centrifugation at 50 g to obtain a sediment of purified hepatocytes [33]. In the work, we used type I collagenase with the activity 146 unit/mg (Amersham Biosciences, UK). Disaggregation of the tissue was performed in a thermostatically Petri dish; a spatula was used to separate cells from the Gleason capsule and vessels. The resulting cell suspension was diluted to 50 ml by Krebs-Ringer bicarbonate buffer containing 0.03% of collagenase, and incubated for 10 min in a thermostat (37°C) upon constant swinging. Further procedures were performed at 4°C. The suspension was filtered twice through gauze to separate nondissociated tissue fragments, cell aggregates, and remnants of connective tissue. Hepatocytes were isolated by centrifugation at 50 g from the filtrate represented by a mixed cell suspension.

Cells count was done in a Goryaev chamber. Viability and purity of cell fractions were estimated using the light microscopy.

Isolation of murine peritoneal macrophages. Experiments were performed on peritoneal macrophages from male A/Sn(A) mice aging 3-4 months and weighing 20-24 g. HA-1 ascitic hepatoma was induced by *o*-aminoazotoluene (Institute of Cytology and Genetics, Siberian Division of the Russian Academy of Sciences, Novosibirsk). Tumor-associated macrophages were harvested from the ascitic fluid due to adgesive properties of cells. Ascitic fluid cells were resuspended in RPMI-1640 medium with 2mM L-glutamine (pH 7.4) containing 20 mM HEPES (ICN Biomedicals, Inc). The cells were incubated in 6-well plates (Orange Scientific) in a CO_2-incubator (Cole-Parmer) at 5% CO_2 (37°C). After 30-min incubation nonadherent cells were removed by 2 times washing with RPMI-1640 medium. Greater than 90% of attached cells were macrophages as determined by light microscopy. The density of tumor-associated macrophages was 1500 cells/mm^2.

Intracellular interleukin-1β assay in the murine peritoneal macrophages. Experiments were performed with bacterial polysaccharides (*E. coli* LPS, Sigma) and yeast polysaccharides (carboxymethylated and sulfoethylated glucans, CMG and SEG; Institute of Chemistry, Slovakian Academy of Sciences). Polysaccharides (10 μg/ml) were added to the macrophage incubation medium. After 2 h incubation the cells were lysed with a solution containing 10 mM sodium phosphate (pH 7.2), 85 mM NaCl, 5 mM KCl, 0.5% sodium deoxycholate, and 1% Triton X-100. Interleukin-1β concentration in the cell lysate was measured by solid-phase enzyme immunoassay using a "ProCon IL1-beta commercial test system" (Russia). The measurements were performed on a Multiscan MCC-340 vertical photometer at 450 nm.

Fluorescence analysis of the interaction for LPS binding to HDL and apoA-I. Tryptophan fluorescence quenching is commonly used to confirm the interaction of a ligand with protein [34]. Fluorescence measurements were performed using a Shimadzu RF-5301 PC (Kyoto, Japan) spectrofluorometer. We determined the fluorescence quenching at interaction of polysaccharides (*E. coli* LPS, Sigma) and yeast polysaccharides (carboxymethylated and sulfoethylated glucans, CMG and SEG; Institute of Chemistry, Slovakian Academy of Sciences) with VLDL, HDL, LDL, and apolipoprotein A-I. Fluorescence was collected from 300 to 550 nm and resulting from a 280 nm excitation.

Preparation of FITC-LPS complexes. LPS were labeled with FITC according to the protocol of Skelly R.S. et al. [35]. FITC-LPS complexes was prepared by incubating 1 mg of LPS and 4 mg of FITC (Sigma Chemical Co.) in 5.0 ml of 0.1 M sodium borate, pH 10.5, for 3 h at 37°C. After incubation, the mixture was dialyzed exhaustively against 0.15 M NaCl for separating free FITC from conjugated FITC-LPS. The concentration of FITC in FITC-LPS was determined at 493 nm. Fluorescence measurements were performed using a Shimadzu RF-5301 PC (Kyoto, Japan) spectrofluorometer.

LPS uptake into hepatocytes using a fluorescence microscopy. For fluorescence microscopy 8 x 10^5 isolated hepatocytes in 1 ml of PBS were incubated with 10 μg/ml FITC labeled LPS in the presense 50 μg apoA-I or without an apoA-I for times up to 30 min. Cells were then washed twice in PBS before fixation with 2% paraformaldehyde. The cells that were suspended in PBS and placed on glass slides. LPS uptake into hepatocytes was visualized using an «AxioImager Z1» (Zeiss, Germany) fluorescence microscopy and quantified using the «AxioCam MRc» digital camera and the software of AxioVision V. 4.5.

Statistical analysis. Analysis of variance was used to test the hypothesis of equality. The results were analyzed by Student´s *t*-test at a significance level of $p \leq 0.05$.

Results

Analysis of Interaction of Blood Plasma Lipoproteins with Bacterial and Yeast Polysaccharides

One of the most informative methods for studying complex formation is fluorescence spectroscopy that makes it possible to detect conformational changes in protein molecule as a result of the formation of an interaction with the ligand. The method is informative due to the difference in spectral characteristics of the complex and free substance. Of the three fluorescent amino acids (tryptophan, tyrosine, phenylalanine) only tryptophan gives more complete information about the structure of the macromolecule and about the character of its microenvironment during complex formation [34].

Our work, using the method of quenching of tryptophane fluorescence, describes binding of high-density lipoproteins (HDL), low-density lipoproteins (LDL) and very low-density lipoproteins (VLDL) to polysaccharides of bacterial and yeast origin. For this aim we used the strongest and well studied inducer of a systemic inflammatory response – a bacterial lipopolysaccharide from *Escherichia coli* (LPS). We also used carboxymethylated (CMG) and sulfoethylated (SEG) D-glucans from the cell wall of *Basidiomycetes* and *Oomycetes*, that possess immune-modulating properties [36]. The interaction of polysaccharides with lipoproteins was accompanied by the change in the spectral characteristics of tryptophan residues that enter into the structure of apolipoproteins. The formation of complexes was judged by the luminous intensity change and fluorescence spectra shift.

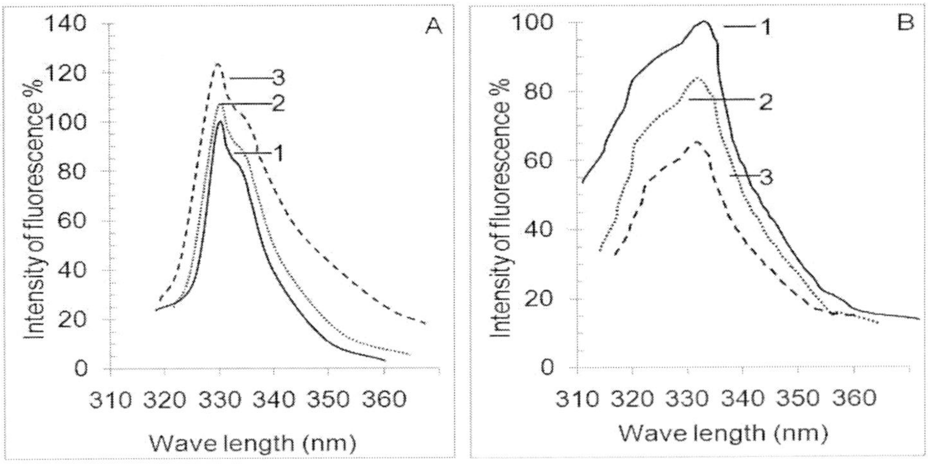

Figure 1. Tryptophan fluorescence quenching of lipoproteins at interaction with polysaccharides (*E. coli* LPS). HDL – (A); LDL – (B). (——) — LP, initial spectrum; (·······) — LP spectrum in the presence LPS after 5 min; (- - - -) — LP spectrum in the presence LPS after 30 min.

The interaction of LPS with lipoproteins was accompanied by the change in tryptophan fluorescence intensity depending on time. Full saturation of the binding areas of lipoprotein particles with lipopolysaccharide was observed 30 minutes after the beginning of the experiment. The interaction of LPS with HDL resulted in a tryptophan fluorescence increase by 25% (Figure 1A), with VLDL – by 10% (data not shown)), and during the interaction with LDL a pronounced fluorescence quenching by 35-40% was observed (Figure 1B).

During the interaction of LPS with lipoproteins the tryptophanyl fluorescence spectra shape remained nearly the same. However, a weak shift by 1-3 nm into the short-wave area was observed, which is explained by the increase of hydrophobicity of the tryptophan environment and local conformational rearrangements of the protein component of lipoprotein particles after its interaction with the ligand.

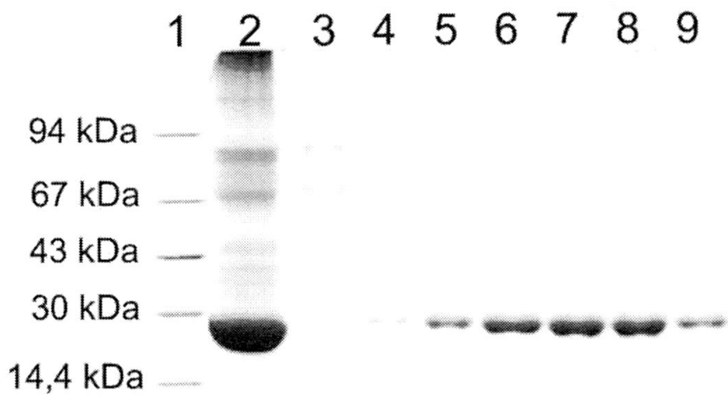

Figure 2. SDS-PAG electrophoregram of chromatographic cleaning of apolipoprotein A-I. Lane 1 - low-molecular weight protein standards: phosphorylase, 94 kDa; albumin, 67 kDa; ovalbumin, 43 kDa; carboanhydrase, 30 kDa; and lactalbumin, 14.4 kDa. Lane 2 - total rat HDL protein. Lanes 3-9 – stages of purity apolipoprotein A-I.

Different directions of changes of spectral characteristics of HDL, LDL and VLDL fluorescence after the formation of their complexes with LPS is explained by the differences in conformational rearrangements of lipoprotein particles and, as a consequence, by the degree of accessibility of tryptophanyls in the water phase for photons.

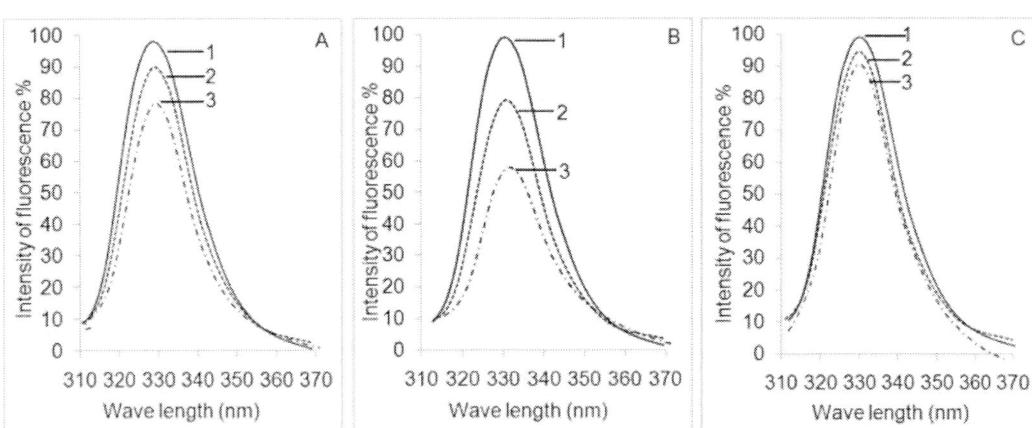

Figure 3. Tryptophan fluorescence quenching of apoA-I at interaction with polysaccharides: LPS – (A); CMG – (B); SEG – (C). (——) — apoA-I, initial spectrum, (- - - - -) — apoA-I spectrum in the presence polysaccharides after 5 min; (- · · - · ·) — apoA-I spectrum in the presence polysaccharides after 30 min.

In order to answer the question about the role of lipid and protein components of lipoproteins in polysaccharide binding, we researched binding of apoA-I, the main protein component of HDL, to the chosen polysaccharides. Figure 2 shows stages of chromatographic cleaning of apolipoprotein A-I.

The interaction of polysaccharides with apoA-I was accompanied by fluorescence quenching of tryptophan. The quenching during the interaction with LPS was 20%, with CMG – 40%, and with SEG – 10% (Figure 3).

Different directions of changes of spectral characteristics of HDL and apoA-I fluorescence after the formation of their complexes with LPS are very much in evidence. The increase of fluorescence intensity in the first case, as it was already noted, is related to higher accessibility of tryptophanyls in the water phase for the photons, and the fluorescence quenching in the second case can be explained by screening of tryptophanyls directly by the lipopolysaccharide or other amino-acid residues of apolipoprotein as a result of protein molecule conformation change.

We also studied the binding of LPS to different classes of lipoproteins by agarose gel electrophoresis. As LPS is a negatively charged structure due to the presence of phosphoric acid residues, its interaction with lipoproteins with the formation of a complex should be accompanied by the increase of electrophoretic migration of lipoprotein particles to the anode.

Figure 4 shows that the addition of LPS to LDL in the concentration of 10 μg/ml had nearly no influence on the electrophoretic mobility of lipoprotein particles (Figure 4A, lanes 1 and 2).

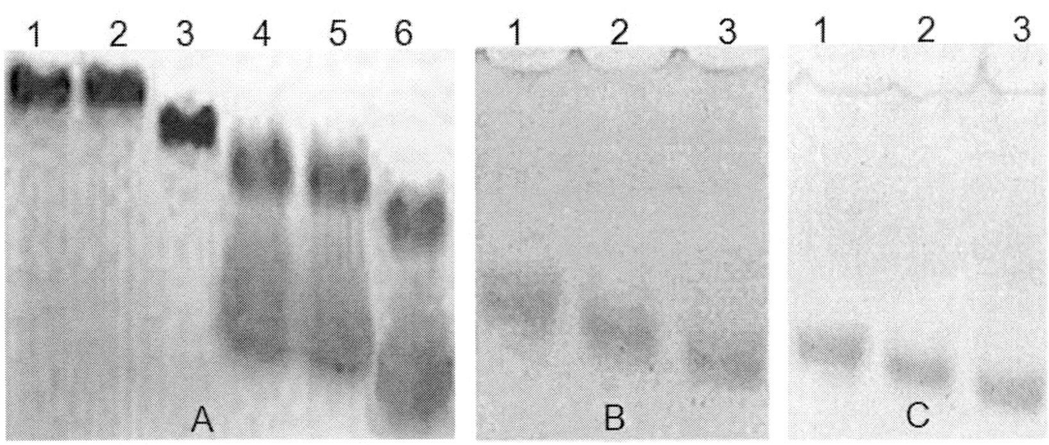

A. Lanes: 1 – LDL (control); 2 – LDL + LPS (10 mg/ml); 3 – LDL + LPS (20 mg/ml; 4 – HDL (control); 5 – HDL + LPS (10 mg/ml); 6 – HDL + LPS (20 mg/ml).
B. Lanes: 1 – VLDL (control); 2 – VLDL + LPS (10 mg/ml); 3 – I VLDL + LPS (20 mg/ml).
C. Lanes: 1 – apoA-I (control); 2 – apoA-I + LPS (10 mg/ml); 3 – apoA-I + LPS (20 mg/ml).

Figure 4. The change of electrophoretic mobility of different lipoproteins and apolipoprotein A-I after interaction with LPS by electrophoresis in 1% agarose gel.

However, when the LPS concentration was 20 μg/ml, LDL mobility increased, which is an evidence of the negative charge increase and modification of the protein component of LDL due to the complex formation (Figure 4A, lane 3). When LPS (10 and 20 μg/ml) was added to HDL (Figure 4A. lanes 4-6) and VLDL (Figure 4B, lanes 2 and 3), their electrophoretic mobility increased proportionally to the amount of the bound LPS. The LPS dose dependent difference in the mobility of HDL-LPS, VLDL-LPS and LDL-LPS complexes is explained by differences in the initial amount of lipoprotein charge. As it is known, LDL are more electropositive due to arginine- and lysine-rich areas. It is these areas that are responsible for the interaction of LDL with B,E-receptors [37].

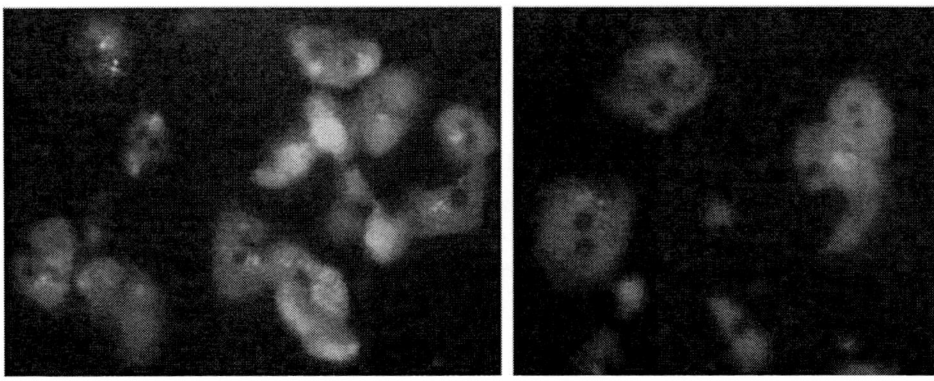

Figure 5. LPS uptake into hepatocytes using a fluorescence microscopy. Isolated hepatocytes were incubated with FITC labeled LPS in the presense apoA-I (A) or without an apoA-I (B).

The same results were obtained during the study of interaction of apoA-I with different concentrations of LPS (10 and 20 μg/ml) on a Figure 4C. Electrophoretic mobility of apoA-I increased proportionally to the amount of the bound LPS, which is a consequence of a decrease the positive charge of the protein molecule as a result of ion interaction with the negatively charged structure of LPS.

Transfer LPS Complexed with apoA-I into Hepatocytes

The ability of apoA-I to bind polysaccharides with the formation of complexes were the grounds for the study of the possibility of intracellular LPS transport by apoA-I. Using isolated hepatocytes of rats and the methods of fluorescence microscopy and spectrofluorimetry we showed the ability of apoA-I to transport LPS into the cell. For this aim we used a FITC labeled LPS. Hepatocytes ($8x10^5$ cells) were incubated with FITC-LPS (10 μg/ml) and with the complex of FITC-LPS-apoA-I for 30 minutes at the temperature of 37°C in serum-free medium so that serum factors able to aid LPS uptake would not interfere with the results. The complex of apoA-I with FITC-LPS was prepared in the molar ratio of 2:1. After the incubation the cells were repeatedly washed with the phosphate-buffered saline (pH 7.4, 4°C), containing 1 mM EDTA-Na_2, and were studied with a fluorescence microscope.

Cell fluorescence (x40 lens magnification) was analyzed in 5 fields of vision of each of the 6 preparations in the study group. Digital cell images were binarized according to brightness and analyzed by means of the *VideoTest Morpho 3.2* software. The average value of the sum of areas ($pixel^2$) of binary images was accepted as the conditional indicator of FITC-LPS content. Visualization of hepatocytes in the regime of fluorescence showed the accumulation of FITC-LPS in the cytoplasm, which was most pronounced during the use of FITC-LPS complexed with apoA-I (Figure 5).

That is demonstrated by the results of digital cell image processing (10 750±473 conditional units versus 3200±280 conditional units in the control, $p<0.001$). The spectrofluorimetric analysis confirmed the microscopy data. Fluorescence intensity of hepatocytes lysates after the incubation with FITC-LPS complexed with apoA-I was higher (83.7±7.15 as compared with 12.7±4.28 in the control, $p<0.001$).

Influence of Lipoproteins and Lipoproteins-bound Polysaccharides on IL-1β Production by Tumor-associated Macrophages

It is known macrophages play an important role in antitumor protection. Cytotoxic activity of these cells is associated with secretion of some cytokines and reactive oxygen metabolites [38, 39]. However, recent studies showed that macrophages are involved in tumor progression. Functional activity of macrophages is modulated by tumor microenvironment: these cells gain the ability to maintain tumor growth, which is realized via stimulation angiogenic activity and increase in the invasive and metastatic potential of the tumor [40 – 42]. Proinflammatory cytokine interleukin-1β (IL-1β) is a regulatory macrophage factor. IL-1β promotes tissue regeneration and stimulates metastatic dissemination during tumor growth [43]. Some attempts were made to neutralize IL-1β in oncological diseases. However, many drugs do not satisfy the demands. In light of this, the search for new products that circulate for a long time and provide a strong therapeutic effect is an important problem. We believe that these properties are typical of plasma lipoproteins.

Chronic inflammation plays an important role in tumor development [44 – 46]. Various polysaccharides, including bacterial lipopolysaccharides (LPS) and yeast carboxymethylated (CMG) or sulfoethylated glycans (SEG), can induce chronic inflammation. Here we studied the effects of HDL, LDL, and their complexes with polysaccharides on IL-1β concentration in peritoneal macrophages from mice with HA-1 ascitic hepatoma.

Table 1. IL-1β concentration in peritoneal macrophages from mice with HA-1 ascitic hepatoma (pg/ml, M±m, n=6)

Additives in the incubation medium	HDL	LDL
No additives	5.3±1.0*	20.2±2.3*
Cortisol	2.3±0.4*	15.4±1.2*
LPS	12.8±1.8*	25.8±2.6*
CMG	16.1±1.0*	30.1±2.8*
SEG	13.5±0.7*	28.0±1.5*

Note: * $p<0.05$ compared to the control.

IL-1β concentration in control samples was 43.3±3.7 pg/ml. Table 1 shows that 2-h incubation of mouse peritoneal macrophages with HA-1 ascitic hepatoma in the presence of lipoproteins (a protein concentration of 1 mg/ml) was followed by a decrease in intracellular IL-1β concentration. These changes were most pronounced in the presence of HDL. Under these conditions, IL-1β concentration decreased by 8 times compared to the control. Our results are consistent with published data [47]. The presence of LDL in the incubation medium was accompanied by a 2-fold decrease in IL-1β concentration.

Glucocorticoids or their synthetic analogues are extensively used as inductors of tumor cell apoptosis in the therapy of tumors [48]. Moreover, glucocorticoids can inhibit the production of proinflammatory factors by macrophages [49, 50]. In our experiments, the effect of cortisol (10^{-6} M) was similar to that of HDL. IL-1β concentration decreased by 9.6 times compared to the control (4.5±0.9 pg/ml, $p<0.05$). Combined treatment of macrophages with HDL and cortisol induced a greater decrease in IL-1β concentration (by 19 times).

We showed that addition of polysaccharides (10μg/ml) in complexes with lipoproteins is followed by a decrease in IL-1β concentration by 1.5-3.0 times compared to the control (Table 1). A complexes of polysaccharides and HDL had the strongest effect. Individual treatment with polysaccharides had no effect on IL-1β concentration in macrophages. Probably, tumor-associated macrophages are primed and cannot induce further increase in the secretion of proinflammatory cytokine. There are similar results in the literature. In particular, it was found that Wiskott-Aldrich syndrome microglia were impaired in production of inflammatory cytokines such as TNF-α, IL-6 and IL-1β upon LPS stimulation [51].

Our observations indicate that lipoproteins can produce an antiinflammatory effect. The mechanism for the action of lipoproteins on functional activity of tumor-associated macrophages remains unknown. Probably, the effect of lipoproteins is related to regulatory properties of their protein components (apolipoproteins). The formation of polysaccharide-lipoproteins complexes in blood plasma serves as a defense mechanism, which reduces the severity of chronic inflammation during tumor growth.

Conclusion

The ability of blood plasma lipoproteins to bind lipopolysaccharide in the Gram-negative bacteria cell wall is well known in the literature. For example, in the papers by Ulevitch R.J. et al. [1, 52], complexes of lipopolysaccharide and lipoproteins of high density were first extracted from rabbit blood plasma and characterized. That marked the beginning of the study of HDL new function that implies their ability to neutralize LPS and thus to produce a protective effect during endotoxemia. Later it was found that lipoproteins of other classes are also able to bind LPS in the blood, and that endotoxin can be transported into the cell by means of receptor-mediated endocytosis in the complexes with LDL [5].

Now it is known, that both protein and lipid components of lipoprotein particles take part in the process of complex formation. ApoA-I as the main protein component of HDL plays an important role in the process of LPS binding [8, 53]. Changes in the apoA-I structure, for example replacement of amino-acid residues, significantly decreases the protective effect of HDL [18]. It is important to note that apoA-I mimetic peptides also produce the protective effect and are able to bind LPS, inhibiting the interaction of endotoxin with lipopolysaccharide binding protein (LBP) [14, 15]. However, the question about competitive relations between apoA-I and LBP remains open to discussion. On the basis of the data available in literature one should not exclude the possibility of formation of a triple complex with the participation of LPS, LBP and apoA-I [8, 9]. The contribution of the lipid component of HDL into LPS binding and implementation of the protective effect of the particles is still not fully understood. Some authors note the absence of the difference in the effects exhibited by apoA-I and HDL [8]. At the same time, other researchers conclude that the degree of manifestation of the HDL protective effect is proportional to the amount of phospholipids, but not of protein components in the particle structure [20].

In this paper, by means of tryptophan fluorescence quenching and agarose gel electrophoresis, we show the ability of lipoproteins (HDL, LDL, VLDL) to bind polysaccharides of different nature: LPS from *Escherichia coli*, as well as glucans from the yeast cell wall. The polysaccharide-lipoprotein complex formation mechanism can be considered as the ligand-receptor interaction. It is noted that the apoA-I protein component of polysaccharides takes part in their interaction with HDL. The properties of polysaccharides of yeast origin have recently been actively studied. For example, the antioxidant, antimutagenic, and antigenotoxic effects of glucans were discovered [36]. Their possible application in anticancer prevention/therapy is under study. In this aspect, the discovered ability of apoA-I to interact with yeast polysaccharides is of great importance, as it suggests direct participation of apoA-I in the implementation of their biological effects. For example, it is possible that these polysaccharides can be transported, including intracellular transport, by means of apoA-I as a carrier.

In this paper we show the ability of apoA-I to increase the efficiency of LPS transport into isolated rat hepatocytes. LPS complexed with apoA-I is transported into the cell through receptor-mediated endocytosis with the possible participation of scavenger receptors. It stands to reason that the intensity of LPS-induced inflammation is inversely proportional to the level of SR-BI expression [30]. The protective effect of HDL and apoA-I against endotoxin is described in numerous studies. However, the mechanism of anti-inflammatory action is not clearly understood. The question about the role of Kupffer cells and hepatocytes in LPS degradation has not been completely solved. The obtained data suggest that the mechanism of anti-inflammatory action of HDL and apoA-I during endotoxemia can be related not only to the inhibition of LPS elimination from the blood with the participation of macrophages, but also to the possibility of metabolic LPS degradation in hepatocytes without the participation of macrophages. This way of endotoxin neutralization can be considered as an alternative and relatively safe way, that makes it possible to reduce the cascade of reactions with the formation of a receptor complex of CD14/TLR4/MD2, activation of NF-κB and induction of the synthesis of pro-inflammatory cytokines. Earlier studies in our laboratory showed that after LPS administration to rats the ability of hepatocytes to uptake HDL increases, and that one of Kupffer cells decreases [54].

As it was already noted, lipoprotein-bound LPS is not able to induce full-scale activation of macrophages. In this paper we show the stronger ability of HDL as compared with LDL and as well of their complexes with polysaccharides of different nature to inhibit the production of pro-inflammatory cytokine with metastatic potential of IL-1β. This effect was shown by means of the model of tumor growth in the culture of tumor-associated macrophages. The pronounced effect of HDL was equal to the anti-inflammatory action of cortisol. The combined use of HDL and cortisol resulted in the additive effect. The obtained results agree with the data of other authors. Thus, HDL and apoA-I-mediated decrease of production of IL-1β and other pro-inflammatory cytokines by monocytes and lymphocytes is shown [47, 55].

Summarizing the obtained results and analyzing data of other authors, we can suggest mechanisms of the anti-inflammatory effect of HDL and apoA-I. On the one hand, they can be conditioned by the participation of apoA-I in the regulation of expression of genes of pro-inflammatory cytokines in macrophages. The influence of HDL on the regulation of activity of the NF-κB nuclear factor is noted in literature [56]. On the other hand, they can be related to the creation of additional ways internalization of polysaccharides into cells with the participation of lipoprotein receptors [57, 58] that exclude the activation of transcription of cytokine cascade genes, for example, scavenger receptors that are present both on hepatocytes and liver macrophages. Thus, in the studies reported here, we have demonstrated that lipoproteins of different classes and apoA-I bind bacterial and yeast polysaccharides and decrease IL-1β production by tumor-associated macrophages (TAMs) and prevent the activation of polysaccharide-treated TAMs. We have also shown that apoA-I can be the LPS carrier into isolated hepatocytes of rat.

References

[1] Ulevitch, R.J., Johnston, A.R., Weinstein, D.B. New function for high density lipoproteins. Isolation and characterization of a bacterial lipopolysaccharide-high density lipoprotein complex formed in rabbit plasma. *J. Clin. Investig*. 1981. 67(3): 827-837.

[2] Navab, M., Hough, G.P., Van Lenten, B.J., Berliner, J.A., Fogelman, A.M. Low density lipoproteins transfer bacterial lipopolysaccharides across endothelial monolayers in a biologically active form. *J. Clin. Invest*. 1988. 81(2): 601-605.

[3] Harris, H.W., Grunfeld, C., Feingold, K.R., Rapp, J.H. Human very low density lipoproteins and chylomicrons can protect against endotoxin-induced death in mice. *J. Clin. Invest.* 1990. 86(3): 696-702.

[4] Feingold, K.R., Funk, J.L., Moser, A.H., Shigenada, J.K., Rapp, J.H., Grunfeld, C. Role for circulating lipoproteins in protection from endotoxin toxicity. *Infect. Immun*. 1995. 63(5): 2041-2046.

[5] Van Lenten, B.J., Fogelman, A.M., Haberland, M.E., Edwards, P.A. The role of lipoproteins and receptor-mediated endocytosis in the transport of bacterial lipopolysaccharide. *Proc. Natl. Acad. Sci. USA*. 1986. 83(8): 2704-2708.

[6] Su, G.L. Lipopolysaccharides in liver injury: molecular mechanisms of Kupffer cell activation. *Am. J. Physiol. Gastrointest. Liver Physiol.* 2002. 283(2): 256-265.

[7] Van Amersfoort, E.S., Van Berkel, T.J., Kuiper, J. Receptors, mediators, and mechanisms involved in bacterial sepsis and septic shock. *Clin. Microbiol. Rev*. 2003. 16(3): 379-414.

[8] Ma, J., Liao, X.L., Lou, B., Wu, M.P. Role of apolipoprotein A-I in protecting against endotoxin toxicity. *Acta Biochim. Biophys. Sin.* (Shanghai). 2004. 36(6): 419-424.

[9] Massamiri, T., Tobias, P.S., Curtiss, L.K. Structural determinants for the interaction of lipopolysaccharide binding protein with purified high density lipoproteins: role of apolipoprotein A-I. *J. Lipid Res.* 1997. 38(3): 516-525.

[10] Birjmohun, R.S., van Leuven, S.I., Levels, J.H., van 't Veer, C., Kuivenhoven, J.A., Meijers, J.C., Levi, M., Kastelein, J.J., van der Poll, T., Stroes, E.S. High-density lipoprotein attenuates inflammation and coagulation response on endotoxin challenge in humans. *Arterioscler. Thromb. Vasc. Biol.* 2007. 27(5): 1153-1158.

[11] Pajkrt, D., Doran, J.E., Koster, F., Lerch, P.G., Arnet, B., van der Poll, T., ten Cate, J.W., van Deventer, S.J. Antiinflammatory effects of reconstituted high-density lipoprotein during human endotoxemia. *J. Exp. Med.* 1996. 184(5): 1601-1608.

[12] Levine, D.M., Parker, T.S., Donnelly, T.M., Walsh, A., Rubin, A.L. In vivo protection against endotoxin by plasma high density lipoprotein. *Proc. Natl. Acad. Sci. USA* 1993. 90(24): 12040-12044.

[13] Hubsch, A.P., Casas, A.T., Doran, J.E. Protective effects of reconstituted high-density lipoprotein in rabbit gram-negative bacteremia models. *J. Lab. Clin. Med.* 1995. 126(6): 548-558.

[14] Zhang, Z., Datta, G., Zhang, Y., Miller, A.P., Mochon, P., Chen, Y.F., Chatham, J., Anantharamaiah, G.M., White, C.R. Apolipoprotein A-I mimetic peptide treatment inhibits inflammatory responses and improves survival in septic rats. *Am. J. Physiol. Heart Circ. Physiol.* 2009. 297(2): 866-873.

[15] Gupta, H., Dai, L., Datta, G., Garber, D.W., Grenett, H., Li Y., Mishra, V., Palgunachari, M.N., Handattu, S., Gianturco, S.H., Bradley, W.A., Anantharamaiah, G.M., White, C.R. Inhibition of lipopolysaccharide-induced inflammatory responses by an apolipoprotein AI mimetic peptide. *Circ. Res.* 2005. 97(3): 236-243.

[16] Usynin, I.F., Tsyrendorzhiev, D.D., Kharkhovski, A.V., Poliakov, L.M., Panin, L.E. Effect of plasma lipoproteins and apolipoprotein A-I on lipopolysaccharide-induced production of reactive oxygen metabolites by Kupffer cells of the rat. *Biokhimiia* 1996. 61(2): 260-265.

[17] Usynin, I.F., Tsyrendorzhiev, D.D., Kharkhovski, A.V., Panin, L.E. High density lipoprotein-3 prevents lipopolysaccharide-induced liver injury in zymosan-pretreated rats. The Immune Consequences of Trauma, Shock and Sepsis. Faist E., editor. Monduzzi Editore, Bologna (Italy). 1997: 559-563.

[18] Wang, Y., Zhu, X., Wu, G., Shen, L., Chen, B. Effect of lipid-bound apoA-I cysteine mutants on lipopolysaccharide-induced endotoxemia in mice. *J. Lipid. Res.* 2008. 49(8): 1640-1645.

[19] Khovidhunkit, W., Kim, M.S., Memon, R.A., Shigenaga, J.K., Moser, A.H., Feingold, K.R., Grunfeld, C. Effects of infection and inflammation on lipid and lipoprotein metabolism: mechanisms and consequences to the host. *J. Lipid. Res.* 2004. 45(7): 1169-1196.

[20] Hara, T., Ishida, T., Kojima, Y., Tanaka, H., Yasuda, T., Shinohara, M., Toh, R., Hirata, K. Targeted deletion of endothelial lipase increases HDL particles with anti-inflammatory properties both in vitro and in vivo. *J. Lipid. Res.* 2011. 52(1): 57-67.

[21] Treon, S.P., Thomas, P., Broitman, S.A. Lipopolysaccharide (LPS) processing by Kupffer cells releases a modified LPS with increased hepatocyte binding and decreased tumor necrosis factor-alpha stimulatory capacity. *Proc. Soc. Exp. Biol. Med.* 1993. 202 (2): 153-158.

[22] Mimura, Y., Sakisaka, S., Harada, M., Sata, M., Tanikawa, K. Role of hepatocytes in direct clearance of lipopolysaccharide in rats. *Gastroenterology* 1995. 109(6): 1969-1976.

[23] Fukuda, I., Tanamoto, K., Kanegasaki, S., Yajima, Y., Goto, Y. Deacylation of bacterial lipopolysaccharide in rat hepatocytes in vitro. *Br. J. Exp. Pathol.* 1989. 70(3): 267-274.

[24] Parent, J.B. Membrane receptors on rat hepatocytes for the inner core region of bacterial lipopolysaccharides. *J. Biol. Chem.* 1990. 265(6): 3455-3461.

[25] Díaz-Laviada, I., Ainaga, J., Portolés, M.T., Carrascosa, J.L., Muncio, A.M., Pagani, R. Binding studies and localization of Escherichia coli lipopolysaccharide in cultured hepatocytes by an immunocolloidal-gold technique. *Histochem. J.* 1991. 23(5): 221-228.

[26] Liu, S., Khemlani, L.S., Shapiro, R.A., Johnson, M.L., Liu, K., Geller, D.A., Watkins, S.C., Goyert, S.M., Billiar, T.R. Expression of CD14 by hepatocytes: upregulation by cytokines during endotoxemia. *Infect. Immun.* 1998. 66(11): 5089-5098.

[27] Vodovotz, Y., Liu, S., McCloskey, C., Shapiro, R., Green, A., Billiar, T.R. The hepatocyte as a microbial product-responsive cell. *J. Endotoxin Res.* 2001. 7(5): 365-373.

[28] Scott, M.J., Billiar, T.R. Beta 2-integrin-induced p38 MAPK activation is a key mediator in the CD14/TLR4/MD2-dependent uptake of lipopolysaccharide by hepatocytes. *J. Biol. Chem.* 2008. 283(43):.29433-29446.

[29] Shao, B., Munford, R.S., Kitchens, R., Varley, A.W. Hepatic uptake and deacylation of the LPS in bloodborne LPS-lipoprotein complexes. *Innate Immun.* 2012. Mar 22. [Epub ahead of print].

[30] Guo, L., Song, Z., Li, M., Wu, Q., Wang, D., Feng, H., Bernard, P., Daugherty, A., Huang, B., Li, X.A. Scavenger Receptor BI protects against septic death through its role in modulating inflammatory response. *J. Biol. Chem.* 2009. 284(30): 19826-19834.

[31] Hatch, F.T. Practical method for plasma lipoprotein analysis. *Adv. Lipid Res.* 1968. 6: 1-68.

[32] Herbert, P.N., Shulman, R.S., Levy, R.I., Fredrickson, D.S. Fractionation of the C-apoproteins from human plasma very low density lipoproteins. *J. Biol. Chem.* 1973. 248(14): 4941-4946.

[33] Seglen, P.O. Preparation of isolated rat liver cells. *Methods Cell Biol.* 1976. 13: 29-83.

[34] Lakovich, J. Principles of fluorescence spectroscopy. Moscow, *Mir.* 1986. 496 p.

[35] Skelly, R.R., Munkenbeck, P., Morrison, D.C. Hapten-lipopolysaccharides without repeating polymeric structure. *Infection and immunity* 1979. 23(1): 287-293.

[36] Kogan, G., Pajtinka, M., Babincova, M., Miadokova, E., Rauko, P., Slamenova, D., Korolenko, T.A. Yeast cell wall polysaccharides as antioxidants and antimutagens: can they fight cancer? *Neoplasma* 2008. 55(5): 387-393.

[37] Triau, J.E., Arbetter, J., Schaefer, E.J. Impaired hepatocyte binding, uptake and degradation of glucosylated low-density lipoproteins. *Biochim. Biophys. Acta* 1986. 877(3): 359-365.

[38] Martin, J.H., Edwards, S.W. Changes in mechanisms of monocyte/macrophage-mediated cytotoxicity during culture. Reactive oxygen intermediates are involved in monocyte-mediated cytotoxicity, whereas reactive nitrogen intermediates are employed by macrophages in tumor cell killing. *J. Immunol.* 1993. 150(8): 3478-3486.

[39] Ross, J.A., Auger, M.J. The biology of the macrophage. In: The macrophage. 2nd ed. Burke B., Lewis C.E., editors. Oxford (United Kingdom): Oxford University Press. 2002.

[40] Elgert, K.D., Alleva, D.G., Mullins, D.W. Tumor-induced immune dysfunction: the macrophage connection. *J. Leukoc. Biol.* 1998. 64(3): 275-290.

[41] Bingle, L., Brown, N.J., Lewis, C.E. The role of tumour-associated macrophages in tumour progression: implications for new anticancer therapies. *J. Pathol.* 2002. 196(3): 254-265.

[42] Lewis, C., Murdoch, C. Macrophage responses to hypoxia. *Am. J. Pathol.* 2005. 167(3): 627-634.

[43] Elaraj, D.M., Weinreich, D.M., Varghese, S., Puhlmann, M., Hewitt, S.M., Carroll, N.M., Feldman, E.D., Turner, E.M., Alexander, H.R. The role of interleukin 1 in growth and metastasis of human cancer xenografts. *Clin. Cancer Res.* 2006. 12(4): 1088-1096.

[44] Coussens, L.M., Werb, Z. Inflammation and cancer. *Nature* 2002. 420(6917): 860-867.

[45] Suganuma, M., Okabe, S., Kurusu, M., Iida, N., Ohshima, S., Saeki, Y., Kishimoto, T., Fujiki, H. Discrete roles of cytokines, TNF-α, IL-1, IL-6 in tumor promotion and cell transformation. *Int. J. Oncol.* 2002. 20(1): 131-136.

[46] Lin, W.W., Karin, M. A cytokine-mediated link between innate immunity, inflammation and cancer. *J. Clin. Invest.* 2007. 117(5): 1175-1183.

[47] Hyka, N., Dayer, J.M., Modoux, C., Kohno, T., Edwards, C.K., Roux-Lombard, P., Burger, D. Apolipoprotein A-I inhibits the production of interleukin-1 beta and tumor necrosis factor-alpha by blocking contact-mediated activation of monocytes by T lymphocytes. *Blood* 2001. 97(8): 2381-2389.

[48] Schmidt, S., Rainer, J., Ploner, C., Presul, E., Riml, S., Kofler, R. Glucocorticoid-induced apoptosis and glucocorticoid resistance: molecular mechanisms and clinical relevance. *Cell Death Differ.* 2004.11(1): 45-55.

[49] Hamalainen, M., Lilja, R., Kankaanranta, H., Moilanen, E. Inhibition of iNOS expression and NO production by anti-inflammatory steroids. Reversal by histone deacetylase inhibitors. *Pulm. Pharmacol. Ther.* 2008. 21(2): 331-339.

[50] Kleiman, A., Hübner, S., Parkitna, J.M. Rodriguez, Neumann, A., Hofer, S., Weigand, M.A., Bauer, M., Schmid, W., Schütz, G., Libert, C., Reichardt, H.M., Tuckermann, J.P. Glucocorticoid receptor dimerization is required for survival in septic shock via suppression of interleukin-1 in macrophages. *FASEB J.* 2012. 26(2): 722-729.

[51] Sato, M., Ogihara, K., Sawahata, R., Sekikawa, K., Kitani, H. Impaired LPS-induced signaling in microglia overexpressing the Wiskott-Aldrich syndrome protein N-terminal domain. *Int. Immunol.* 2007. 19(8): 901-911.

[52] Ulevitch, R.J., Johnston. A.R., Weinstein. D.B. New function for high density lipoproteins. Their participation in intravascular reactions of bacterial lipopolysaccharides. *J. Clin. Invest.* 1979. 64(5): 1516-1524.

[53] Emancipator, K., Csako, G., Elin, R.J. In vitro inactivation of bacterial endotoxin by human lipoproteins and apolipoproteins. *Infect. Immun.* 1992. 60(2): 596-601.

[54] Usynin, I.F., Panin, L.E., Kharkovski, A.V., Gorjacheva M.V., Ostanina, L.S., Trubitsina, O.M., Tretjakova, T.A. Effect of activation of the mononuclear phagocyte system on hepatic lipoprotein synthesis and plasma lipoprotein binding to rat hepatocytes, Kupffer and endothelial cells. In: Cells of the hepatic sinusoid. Wisse E., Knook D.L., Wake K., editors. The Kupffer cell Foundation, Leiden, the Netherlands. 1995. 5: 297-298.

[55] De Sanctis, J.B., Blanca, I., Bianco, N.E. Secretion of cytokines by natural killer cells primed with interleukin-2 and stimulated with different lipoproteins. *Immunology*. 1997. 90(4): 526-533.

[56] Park, S.H., Park, J.H., Kang, J.S., Kang, Y.H. Involvement of transcription factors in plasma HDL protection against TNF-alpha-induced vascular cell adhesion molecule-1 expression. *Int. J. Biochem. Cell. Biol*. 2003. 35(2): 168-182.

[57] Fidge, N.H. High density lipoprotein receptors, binding proteins, and ligands. *J. Lipid. Res*. 1999. 40(2): 187-201.

[58] Van Oosten, M., van Amersfoort, E.S., van Berkel, T.J., Kuiper, J. Scavenger receptor-like receptors for the binding of lipopolysaccharide and lipoteichoic acid to liver endothelial and Kupffer cells. *J. Endotoxin Res*. 2001. 7(5): 381-384.

In: Apolipoproteins
Editors: A. D. Sidorov and M. Y. Nikitin
ISBN: 978-1-62257-484-1

Chapter VI

Apolipoprotein A-I Motifs in Discoidal High Density Lipoproteins Influence Lecithin: Cholesterol Acyltransferase Activity

Alexander D. Dergunov [*]
National Research Centre for Preventive Medicine, Moscow, Russia

Abstract

Major output of the numerous studies of LCAT activity toward HDL with apoA-I is restricted by only two and bulk values. Moreover, the contributions of LCAT binding to HDL surface and apoA-I structure to LCAT action at interface have not been evaluated. In the present study cholesterol is considered as alcoholic nucleophile that increases the solvolysis rate of acyl-LCAT intermediate. A complete set of individual rate constants for the formation of acyl-enzyme intermediate (k_2), its hydrolysis/solvolysis by water (k_3) and cholesterol (k_4) may be derived from a full kinetic equation that describes the interface velocity in terms of the initial surface concentrations of phosphatidylcholine and cholesterol in discoidal HDL. This analysis was applied to discover the contribution of 139-170 central region of apoA-I molecule to LCAT activation by apolipoprotein. LCAT binding to individual preparations of HDL with Δ139-170 apoA-I deletion mutant or plasma apoA-I was measured with a solid phase assay. The raw kinetic data of Holvoet et al. (Biochemistry (1995) 34: 13334-13342) for these HDL preparations were fitted also with model dependencies of on k_4 within wide range of k_2 and k_3 values. The 139-170 region in apoA-I sequence influences mainly the proper positioning of cholesterol molecule toward LCAT active center, local arginine residue(s) is suggested to contribute primarily. The analysis may be extended for other apoA-I mutations affecting LCAT activity.

Keywords: apolipoprotein; lecithin:cholesterol acyltransferase; apolipoprotein structure

[*] Correspondence: Tel: +7 495 627-0324; Fax: +7 495 628-0094; Email: dergunov@img.ras.ru.

Abbreviations

apoA-I - apolipoprotein A-I;
CE - cholesteryl ester;
Chol – cholesterol;
DPPC – dipalmitoylphosphatidylcholine;
HDL - high density lipoproteins;
LCAT - lecithin:cholesterol acyltransferase;
PC – phosphatidylcholine;
RCT - reverse cholesterol transport;
WT apoA-I – wild-type apoA-I; Δ139-170 apoA-I – apoA-I with a deletion 139-170;

1. Introduction

Atheroprotective role of high-density lipoproteins (HDL) and apolipoprotein (apo) A-I as a major protein constituent of HDL is determined by their contribution into reverse cholesterol transport (RCT) from cells to the liver. RCT efficiency is controlled sequentially by cellular cholesterol (Chol) efflux promoted by lipid-depleted apoA-I and ABCA1 transporter, lipid binding, generation of nascent discoidal HDL as an interface for cholesteryl ester (CE) formation by lecithin:cholesterol acyltransferase (LCAT) and HDL maturation into spherical particle able to interact with cellular receptors and lipid-transport proteins [1]. ApoA-I is a most efficient activator of LCAT and many apolipoprotein coding sequence mutations are associated with poor enzyme activation [2]. The highest LCAT activity has been registered with nascent discoidal HDL [3], which are able to accumulate a limited quantity of cholesteryl ester molecules [4] while spherical HDL particle possess a lower substrate efficiency. Lipid-binding activity of apoA-I, with N- and C-terminal domains that include residues 1-189 and 190-243 [5], respectively, is determined by α-helices differing in sequence position, relative content and orientation of hydrophobic and charged residues. The exact number of α-helices, their position relative phospholipid phase in lipid-bound apoA-I and molecular models of discoidal HDL are presently under investigation [6-12]. The contribution of apolipoprotein domain structure and specific amino acid residues to LCAT activation remains an active area, the lack of LCAT crystallographic structure being a major drawback. The structure of apolipoprotein in lipid-bound state may influence LCAT activity via enzyme binding with the lipid interface, substrate and enzyme activation [13]. Both N- and C-terminal domains seemed to activate LCAT [14]. The low lipid affinity of 144-186 region has been suggested to be important in LCAT activation with the displacement of two apolipoprotein helices from lipid phase by the enzyme molecule and induction of open substrate state [15]. In addition, Sorci-Thomas et al. [16] suggested that LCAT amino acids at position 121–136 may interact with lipid-bound ApoA-I within helix 6 amino acids at position 143–164. However, the direct LCAT-apoA-I interaction, although predicted [17], has not been described yet. The involvement of arginine residues of apoA-I into LCAT activation through enzyme positioning on HDL surface [18] remains to be confirmed and may be otherwise associated with Arg-Chol interaction [19] or more subtle disordering effect of arginine residues on apolipoprotein structure [20;21]. Major output of the numerous studies of

LCAT activity toward HDL with apoA-I (reviewed in [3;22]) is restricted by only two and bulk values. Moreover, the contribution of LCAT binding to HDL surface, an initial step in this interfacial reaction, to the raw kinetic parameters has not been evaluated. In our recent studies [23;24] cholesterol was considered as alcoholic nucleophile that increases the solvolysis rate of acyl-LCAT and a full kinetic analysis of LCAT activity toward discoidal HDL with a fixed or varying apoA-I:phosphatidylcholine (PC) ratio was done. Here this analysis was applied to discover the contribution of apoA-I 139-170 central motif to LCAT activity. Earlier discoidal HDL with this apoA-I deletion mutant has been shown to be a much less efficient substrate compared to HDL with plasma apoA-I [25]. In the present study a quantitative examination of LCAT binding to these HDLs has been performed. The interfacial modeling of raw kinetic data of Holvoet et al. [25] permitted to conclude that 139-170 region in apoA-I sequence influences mainly the proper orientation of cholesterol molecule toward the enzyme active center. The data were compared also with the existing data on the relation of known apoA-I mutations with LCAT activity.

2. Materials and Methods

2.1. Materials

Dipalmitoylphosphatidylcholine (DPPC) and cholesterol were purchased from Sigma (MO, USA). Plasma apoA-I was isolated from delipidated high-density lipoproteins [26]. Wild type (WT) apoA-I and deletion mutant Δ139-170 apoA-I were expressed in E. coli and purified [25]. The purity of apolipoproteins checked by SDS-PAGE was greater than 95%. LCAT was isolated from human plasma [25]; the content of LCAT protein in a crude LCAT preparation did not exceed 20% and contaminants, as detected by SDS-PAGE, consisted of albumin, apoA-I, apoA-IV and low molecular proteins.

2.2. Methods

2.2.1. Preparation and Characterization of Apolipoprotein/DPPC/Chol Complexes

Discoidal reconstituted HDL (rHDL) were prepared and isolated as described [25]. The final apoA-I:DPPC:Chol molar ratios were 1:110:10 for plasma apoA-I and WT apoA-I and 1:80:12 for Δ139-170 apoA-I. Complexes with plasma apoA-I and WT apoA-I contained two apolipoprotein molecules while complex with Δ139-170 apoA-I contained four molecules [25].

2.2.2. rHDL-LCAT Binding Assay

LCAT preparation was immobilized on BrCN-activated Sepharose 4B (Pharmacia, Sweden) according to manufacturer instructions. 1.23 mg of crude LCAT preparation was taken into the reaction, the coupling efficiency and stoichiometry were 61% and 442 μg/ml packed gel, respectively.

The binding was performed in 0.01 M Tris-HCl, pH 8.0, 0.15 M NaCl, 1 mM NaN_3, 0.01% EDTA in a total volume 500 μl with a constant amount of LCAT-Sepharose or Sepharose 4B (20% gel slurry) and different concentrations of rHDL.

After incubation, both sets of tubes were centrifuged and 100 μl buffer were added to 350 μl of supernatant. Second centrifugation was performed to sediment residual gel granules.

Twenty μl of 10% SDS were added to 400 μl of supernatant and samples were incubated at 37 °C for 4 hours. Protein was measured by fluorescence with excitation at 280 nm and emission at 333 nm.

2.2.3. Kinetic Model

The full kinetic analysis of LCAT activity toward discoidal HDL with a fixed and varying POPC and Chol content has been done previously [23;24]. Briefly, two events underlie the kinetic mechanism of cholesteryl ester formation by LCAT: 1) the existence of two consecutive equilibriums, i.e. enzyme binding to the particle (penetration) and LCAT reaction with phosphatidylcholine and cholesterol; 2) this reaction at water-lipid interface proceeds through three steps that involve the formation of acyl-enzyme intermediate and cholesterol as a nucleophilic agent can compete with water at the deacylation of acyl-enzyme (Scheme 1).

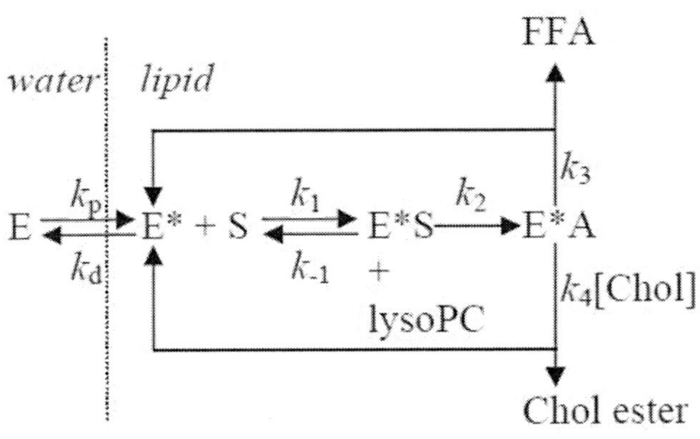

(1)

With this scheme, the bulk/interface expression (Eq. 2) of the velocity v_o/v_i of LCAT-catalyzed cholesteryl ester formation in discoidal HDL at steady state has been derived [23]:

$$\frac{v_o}{[E_t]} = \frac{v_i}{[E_t]} \cdot \frac{I}{V} = \frac{\dfrac{k_2 \cdot k_4 \cdot [Chol]}{k_2 + k_3 + k_4 \cdot [Chol]} \cdot \dfrac{I}{V} \cdot [S]}{\dfrac{k_3 + k_4 \cdot [Chol]}{k_2 + k_3 + k_4 \cdot [Chol]} \cdot K_m^* \cdot \left(K_d^* + \dfrac{I}{V} \right) + \dfrac{I}{V} \cdot [S]}, \tag{2}$$

where $[E_t]$ is the total enzyme concentration (mol/volume); I is the total interfacial area (surface) and V the total volume (volume); v_i is the interface expression of the velocity (mol/surface·time) and v_o is the bulk expression of the rate ((mol/volume·time); k_2 is (time^{-1}); k_3 (time^{-1}); k_4 is the second order rate constant (mol/surface)$^{-1}$(time^{-1}).

Also, is a product k_4·[Chol]. Finally, (*I*/*V*) is the factor for conversion from surface units to bulk units. Surface ([*S*], mol/surface) and bulk ([S_o], mol/volume) substrate (phosphatidylcholine) concentrations are related by Eq. 3:

$$[S] = [S_o]/(I/V). \tag{3}$$

K_m^* and are the interfacial Michaelis-Menten and dissociation constants given by Eq. 4 and 5, respectively:

$$K_m^* = \frac{k_{-1} + k_2}{k_1}, \tag{4}$$

$$K_d^* = \frac{k_d}{k_p} = K_d \cdot area_{LCAT} \cdot 10^{-14} \cdot N_A, \tag{5}$$

where k_p is the penetration rate constant (volume/surface)(time^{-1}); k_d is the desorption rate constant (time^{-1}); k_1 (mol/surface)$^{-1}$(time^{-1}); k_{-1} (time^{-1}); K_d is the dissociation constant of LCAT/disc complex in bulk units (mol/cm^3), $area_{LCAT}$ is the accessible area of LCAT interface recognition region (nm^2), N_A – **Avogadro' number.** K_d should be measured independently. The $area_{LCAT}$ value calculated with the RVP-net web server [27] for the region between 50 and 74 residues in LCAT sequence, suggested to be involved in interfacial recognition [28], was 6.6 nm^2.

The interfacial substrate and cholesterol concentrations (mol·cm^{-2}) are determined by equations 6 and 7, respectively:

$$[S] = \frac{n_{PC} \cdot 10^{14}}{(area_{PC} \cdot n_{PC} + area_{Chol} \cdot n_{Chol}) \cdot N_A} \tag{6}$$

$$[Chol] = \frac{n_{Chol} \cdot 10^{14}}{(area_{PC} \cdot n_{PC} + area_{Chol} \cdot n_{Chol}) \cdot N_A} \tag{7}$$

where n_{PC} and n_{Chol} are the number of PC and Chol molecules per disc and $area_{PC}$ and $area_{Chol}$ are the phosphatidylcholine and cholesterol surface area (nm^2). The values for molecular surface area $area_{PC}$ and $area_{Chol}$ were chosen as 0.46 [29] and 0.38 [30] nm^2, respectively. Thus, the hydrolysis/solvolysis of acyl-LCAT intermediate on the surface of discoidal HDL by water and cholesterol predicts a dependence of CE formation rate on three variables: the surface substrate concentration [*S*], the surface cholesterol concentration [*Chol*] and the proportion of interface *I*/*V*. The apparent catalytic rate constant and Michaelis constant are defined by Eq. 8 and 9, respectively:

$$k_{cat}^{app} = \frac{k_2 \cdot k_4 \cdot [Chol]}{k_2 + k_3 + k_4 \cdot [Chol]} \tag{8}$$

$$K_m^{app} = \frac{k_3 + k_4 \cdot [Chol]}{k_2 + k_3 + k_4 \cdot [Chol]} \cdot K_m^* \cdot \left(K_d^* + \frac{I}{V} \right) \tag{9}$$

In complexes with a constant phosphatidylcholine content (case 1), the value did not vary at the increase of Chol content. Moreover, the apparent decrease of value at the increase of phosphatidylcholine content in complexes with a fixed cholesterol content (case 2) and a concomitant increase of surface area has been shown to originate from the decrease of K_m^*; the *I*/*V* and values contributed oppositely [24]. Consequently, any variation in may be adjusted taking into consideration *I*/*V*, and values. This adjustment is possible if kinetic measurements are performed with a set of complexes of a particular protein, referred above (case 1 or case 2). However, in comparative studies of substrate properties of complexes with different apolipoproteins, measurements are restricted to single complexes that precluded complete kinetic analysis. Nevertheless, some useful considerations are still possible with undefined value. At zero cholesterol, the ratio of kinetic constants (Eq. 10) may be derived from Equation 9:

$$\frac{\frac{k_2}{k_3} + 1}{K_m^*} = \frac{K_d^* + \frac{I}{V}}{K_m^{app}} \tag{10}$$

The value of k_2/k_3 ratio was close to 1 for complexes described by case 1 [23] and the numerator in the left side of equation 10 is suggested to be sensitive to variation of k_2 and k_3 constants. This permits the comparison of individual kinetic constants for LCAT activity toward complexes with different proteins if K_d and values were independently measured. To conclude on the contribution of k_2 and k_3 into k_{cat}^{app}, the dependence of the apparent catalytic rate constant on was modeled by Eq. 11:

$$k_{cat}^{app} = \frac{k_2 \cdot k_4'}{k_2 + k_3 + k_4'} \tag{11}$$

2.2.4. The Influence of Altered ApoA-I Structure on LCAT Activity

The existing data on LCAT activity with natural and/or engineered apoA-I mutations were analyzed in relation to mutation position in apolipoprotein sequence and location in the putative helical segment(s) and to substrates used in the activity assays. Four different substrates were used, i.e. reconstituted discoidal HDLs (D) with individual plasma, wild type and mutant apoA-I; phosphatidylcholine/cholesterol proteoliposomes (L) with a fixed or varying apolipoprotein content in the reaction mixture; isolated plasma HDL (H) or a whole plasma (P). The first approach permits to calculate both and values while only maximal velocity may be derived with a second approach. With the third and fourth approaches, the cholesterol esterification rate (CER) as a measure of endogenous LCAT activity is usually measured. CER, which may be influenced by difference in LCAT mass between two samples and/or heterogeneous nature of lipoprotein substrate, possesses only limited significance in meta-analysis. In all four cases, the change in the kinetic parameter for mutant relative to those for plasma and/or wild type proteins was considered.

3. Results

3.1. Influence of ApoA-I Structure on LCAT Activity

Meta-analysis of natural and engineered apoA-I mutations that affected LCAT activity both in vivo and in vitro included 58 single/double/frame shift mutations and deletions (Table 1). The subset of the data with reconstituted discoidal HDL (D) with individual mutant and native apolipoprotein as substrate (33 mutations affected all residues 1-243) permits to evaluate the effect of altered apolipoprotein structure on the enzyme activity. The data with three other substrates, available as maximal activation only (with proteoliposomes (L)) or cholesterol esterification rate (CER), unadjusted for specific LCAT activity (with HDL (H) and plasma (P)), are included for comparative purpose only. With a five-fold isolated change as a threshold for the effect of altered apoA-I structure on maximal reaction velocity, two non-overlapping regions in the central part and C-domain of apoA-I molecule were involved. They included 139-164 and 190-243 sequences in helices 5-6 and 8-10, respectively. The ranking by maximal activation and CER with L and H/P substrates, respectively, largely confirm this conclusion. Note the prominent response to the replacement of three arginine residues R149, R153 and R160 but only R160 replacement resulted in isolated profound decrease in V_{max}^{app}. Again, the change in two non-overlapping regions in N-domain resulted in isolated increase, i.e. Ser36Ala point mutation in the region between G*-helix and helix 1 (or in helix A by X-ray structure [6]) and Δ63-73 deletion in helices 1-2 (Table 1).

Table 1. The effects of altered apoA-I structure on LCAT activity

Mutation/deletion	Helix	substrate	CER*,%	V_{max}^{app} *,%	K_m^{app} *,%	Ref.
Δ1-43	G*	D		50	186	[31]
Δ1-65	G*-1	D		34	55	[31]
Ser36Ala		D		117	589	[32]
Δ44-126	1-5	D		44	79	[25]
Δ61-78	1-2	D		102	220	[33]
Δ63-73	1-2	D		93	500	[34]
Δ89-99	3	D		58	80	[33]
Asp102Ala/Asp103Ala	4	D		70	136	[35]
Glu110Ala/Glu111Ala	4	D		33	100	[36]

Mutation/deletion	Helix	substrate	CER*,%	V_{max}^{app} *,%	K_m^{app} *,%	Ref.
Δ121-164	5-6	D		20	139	[37]
Δ123-166(A-I), ∇12-75(A-II)	5-6	D		5	139	[38]
Δ139-170	5-7	D		7	79	[25]
140-150 → 63-73	5-6	D		14	571	[34]
Δ140-150	5-6	D		20	429	[34]
Pro143Ala	6	D		30	429	[34]
Pro143Arg	6	D		58	150	[15]
Δ143-164	6	D		14	346	[37]
143-164→220-241	6	D		14	235	[37]
144-164→164-144	6	D		26	132	[37]
Δ144-165	6-7	D		11	2455	[35]
Arg149Gln	6	D		7	38	[18]
Arg149Val	6	D		32	114	[34]
Arg151Cys	6	D		100	150	[39]
Arg153Gln	6	D		9	31	[18]
Val156Glu	6	D		6	644	[40]
Val156Lys	6	D		9	689	[41]
Asp157Lys	6	D		55	267	[41]
Ala158Glu	6	D		15	667	[41]
Arg160Leu	6	D		8	1125	[15]
Arg160Gln	6	D		16	164	[18]
Arg160Leu	6	D		61	84	[42]
Arg160Val/His162Ala	6	D		4	700	[35]
Pro165Arg	7	D		60	145	[42]
Δ190-243	8-10	D		10	93	[25]
Δ190-243(A-I), ∇12-77(A-II)	8-10	D		78	89	[38]
Δ165-175	7	H	27			[43]
Δ44-65	1	L		61		[44]
Δ66-87	2	L		9		[44]
Δ88-98	3	L		49		[44]
Pro99His	4	L	92			[45]
Δ99-120	4	L		15		[44]
Lys107→0	4	L		42		[46]
Lys107→0	4	L		107		[47]
Δ113-124	4-5	L	47			[45]
Pro121His	5	L	77			[45]
Δ121-142	5	L		25		[44]
Pro143Arg	6	L		60		[48]
Δ143-164	6	L		3		[44]

Mutation/deletion	Helix	substrate	CER*,%	V_{max}^{app} *,%	K_m^{app} *,%	Ref.
Δ148-186	6-7	L	0.5			[45]
Leu159Arg	6	L		40		[49]
Δ165-186	7	L		2		[44]
Δ187-208	8	L		7		[44]
Δ209-219	9	L		12		[44]
Δ212-233	9-10	L	28			[45]
Δ213-243	9-10	L	13			[45]
Δ220-241	10	L		17		[44]
Δ100-143	4-5	P	72			[50]
Leu141Arg	5	P	51			[51]
Leu144Arg	6	P	100			[52]
Val156Glu	6	P	50			[53]
Leu159Pro	6	P	64			[54]
FS 162-207 / Δ208-243	6-8	P	26			[55]
Δ165-175	7	P	44			[43]
FS 203-229 / Δ230-243	8-10	P	20			[56]

Substrate: D - discoidal HDL; H - plasma HDL; L - proteoliposome; P – plasma. *) relative values compared to those for WT and/or plasma apoA-I.

Both and values may change thus resulting in the increased for mutant apolipoprotein. Thus, several helical regions in apoA-I structure ultimately affect LCAT activity. However, the use of the apparent kinetic parameters does not permit to evaluate the individual contributions of LCAT binding to HDL surface, the stability of the enzyme-substrate complex and mode of enzyme activation. To separate these events, Δ139-170 apoA-I was studied in more details.

3.2. LCAT Binding to rHDL with Plasma and Δ139-170 apoA-I

The contribution of rHDL-LCAT interaction into enzyme catalytic efficiency was followed by measurements of rHDL binding to immobilized LCAT. The binding parameters of plasma apoA-I/DPPC/Chol and Δ139-170/DPPC/Chol discoidal complexes were compared. The binding kinetics was measured at 6 °C with the lowest disk concentration (Figure 1a). The equilibrium was achieved after 65 hours. The initial attempt to perform the binding reaction at 37 °C did not succeed due to residual LCAT activity. The binding parameters were calculated from Scatchard plots of the data (Figure 1b). For complexes with plasma and apoA-I deletion mutant, the mean K_d values were 64 and 173 nM of apoA-I, respectively. These values roughly coincide if adjusted for different protein stoichiometry, i.e. 2 and 4 protein molecules per rHDL with plasma and apoA-I deletion mutant, respectively. In addition, a four-fold decrease of K_d value for rHDL with plasma apoA-I and DPPC compared to that for rHDL with apoA-I and egg yolk phosphatidylcholine [57], may reflect the lower assay temperature in our study (6 vs. 37 °C) and/or the influence of phosphatidylcholine saturation on LCAT binding [58]. The K_d values expressed as molar concentrations of apoA-I were used in all subsequent calculations. The maximum numbers of binding sites did not differ and equaled 2.18 nmol A-I/mg protein and 2.22 nmol Δ139-170/mg protein, respectively. If 60 kDa M_r value were assumed for the crude protein, the interaction stoichiometry would correspond 1 mol apolipoprotein : 7.6 mol crude protein or 1 mol apoA-I : 1 mol LCAT. In turn, the latter ratio corresponds to 1 rHDL : 2 LCAT and 1 rHDL : 4 LCAT molar ratios for binding of complexes with plasma and deletion mutant apolipoprotein.

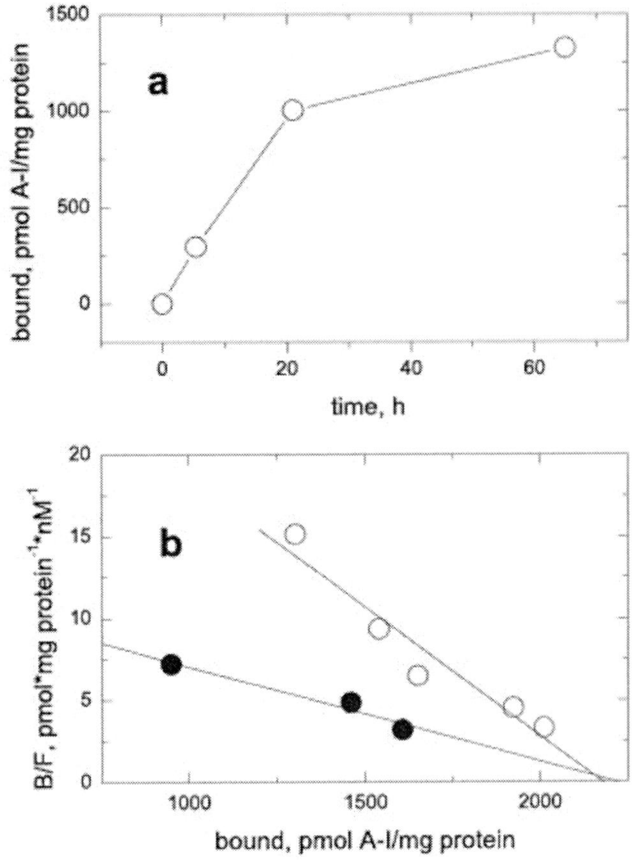

Figure 1. Binding of rHDL with apoA-I proteins to LCAT-Sepharose. (**a**), the kinetics of binding of rHDL with plasma apoA-I; (**b**), Scatchard analysis of the binding of rHDL with plasma apoA-I (open circles) and Δ139-170 apoA-I (closed circles). Data were fitted by linear regression $y = a + b*x$. For rHDL with plasma apoA-I, $a = 34.3 \pm 4.3$, $b = -0.016 \pm 0.003$, $r = -0.96$ ($p = 0.008$); for rHDL with apoA-I deletion mutant, $a = 12.8 \pm 1.6$, $b = -0.006 \pm 0.001$, $r = -0.98$ ($p = 0.13$).

However, the binding stoichiometry may be essentially influenced by complex dimensions, thereby reflecting the increased steric hindrance at the binding of larger rHDL with Δ139-170 apoA-I as compared to plasma protein. LCAT-rHDL interaction may be more accurately described by one-to-one stoichiometry in accordance with others [57].

3.3. LCAT Activity with Native and Δ139-170 Apolipoproteins

The raw data of Holvoet et al. [25] on apparent kinetic parameters and particle composition for discoidal complexes of plasma apoA-I, wild type apoA-I and Δ139-170 apoA-I with DPPC and Chol with different apolipoprotein content per disc were analyzed. The input parameters used in the subsequent calculations are listed in Table 2. The complexes of plasma and wild type apolipoproteins with DPPC and Chol possessed the same lipid area per disc and substrate (DPPC) concentration as complexes with POPC [23]. However, the values for two complexes of plasma and wild type apolipoproteins (0.14 s^{-1}) adjusted for Chol content were 5-fold lower those for complex with POPC (0.7 s^{-1}). Oppositely, values were 5-fold higher for complexes with saturated phosphatidylcholine. The increase in interfacial Michaelis constant with the opposite decrease of interfacial dissociation constant derived from binding experiments for complexes with DPPC (2.5 cm^{-1}) as compared to that for complex with POPC (12 cm^{-1}) [24] may underlie this effect. In turn, the proportion of interface *I*/*V* calculated from bulk value increased for two complexes with DPPC (Table 2). Complexes with Δ139-170 apoA-I possessed the increased surface area compared to those with plasma and wild type apolipoprotein (Table 2) and the interfacial Chol concentration increased 1.6-fold. However, the derived from the bulk K_d value, the latter being expressed as apoA-I level, substantially increased. The difference disappeared if particle concentration was used in the calculation. In accordance with the observations for complexes with POPC [24], the increase of the proportion of interface *I*/*V* for complex with the deletion mutant originated from the decrease of the bulk value.

Table 2. Compositional and kinetic properties of three discoidal reconstituted HDLs

	Apolipoprotein		
	plasma apoA-I	WT apoA-I	Δ139-170 apoA-I
I (nm^2)	109	109	165
DPPC×10^{10} (mol cm^{-2})	3.36	3.36	3.21
Chol×10^{11} (mol cm^{-2})	3.05	3.05	4.82
V_{max}^{app} (nmol CE/h)	6.0	6.2	0.44
K_m^{app} ×10^8 (mol DPPC cm^{-3})	13.2	15.4	7.3
K_d^* (cm^{-1})	2.5	2.5	6.9
I/V (cm^{-1})	393	393	625
$\frac{\frac{k_2}{k_3}+1}{K_m^*}$ ×10^{-9} (mol^{-1} cm^2)	3.0	2.6	8.6

The raw data for complex composition and for apparent kinetic constants [25] were transformed as input values in Equations 8 and 9. Errors are ± 10%. values were calculated from the bulk K_d and the area of LCAT interface recognition region. *I*/*V* values were calculated from the for the complex with plasma apoA-I adjusted for DPPC concentration and disc surface. The ratio of kinetic constants was calculated with Eq. 10.

The adjusted for Chol and surface area value for LCAT activity towards complexes with deletion mutant relative to that for complexes with plasma and wild type apolipoprotein dropped 14-fold. The three k_2, k_3 and k_4 rate constants contribute into (Eq. 8). However, the drop in for LCAT activity towards complexes with Δ139-170 apoA-I was primarily due to drop in k_4, as the $(k_2/k_3+1)/K_m^*$ ratios were comparable for all three complexes taking into account *I/V* change and the expected decrease in for complexes with deletion mutant. Thus, modeling – k'_4 dependencies by equation 11 for three fixed k_2/k_3 ratios (Figure 2) assumes k'_4(Δ139-170 apoA-I) = 0.07 k'_4(plasma/wild type apoA-I). It should be emphasized that previously determined – k'_4 pairs [24] for eight complexes of plasma apoA-I with POPC (Figure 2) fit well this model.

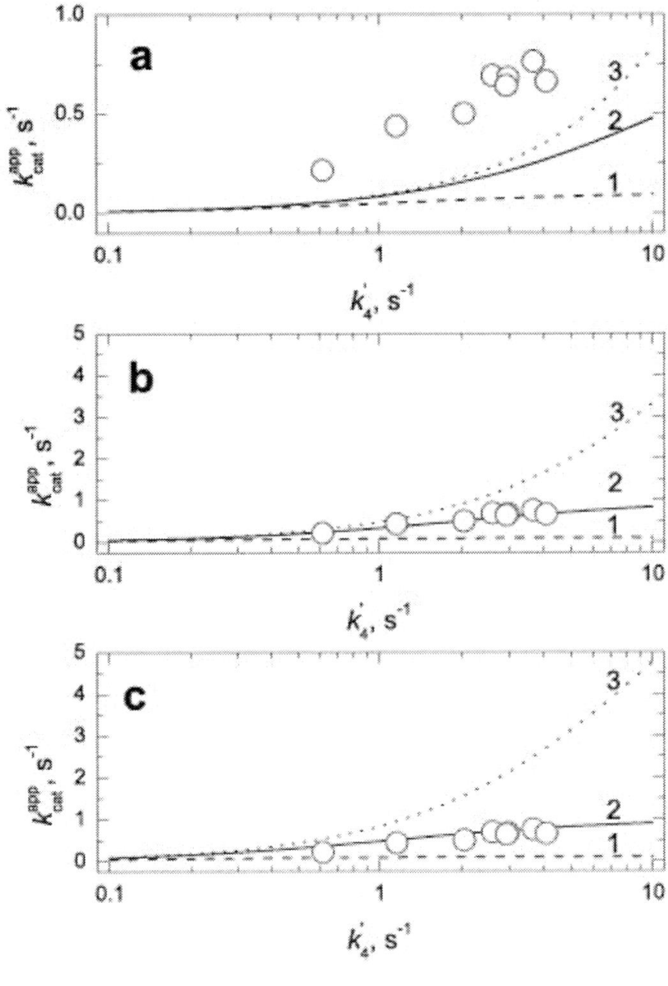

Figure 2. The contribution of acyl-enzyme formation and its hydrolysis by water into LCAT-catalyzed cholesteryl ester formation in discoidal HDL. The dependencies of on were modeled (Eq. 11) with three k_2/k_3 ratios: 0.1 (a), 1.0 (b) and 10.0 (**c**). In each case, calculations were performed with three k_2 values: 0.1 (*1*), 1.0 (*2*) and 10.0 s^{-1} (*3*). The values for eight preparations of HDL with two molecules of apoA-I and POPC with a fixed or varying POPC:apoA-I ratio were also included for comparison.

Discussion

There are three major novelties in the present study. Firstly, the value for complexes of plasma and wild type apoA-I with DPPC significantly decreased compared to that with POPC. LCAT binding to rHDL with egg yolk phosphatidylcholine [3] and various unsaturated synthetic phosphatidylcholines [58] was measured by others. Together, these results suggest the influence of the structure and/or dynamics of the matrix lipid phase of rHDL on LCAT interfacial binding.

Secondly, the lower values for complexes of plasma and wild type apoA-I with DPPC compared to that for complex with POPC with identical PC and Chol surface concentrations is determined by PC fatty acyl composition. Indeed, the decrease in LCAT activity was significantly correlated with a decrease in the fluidity of rHDL prepared with unsaturated PCs [59]. The DPPC bilayer compared to those from unsaturated PCs is much more rigid at the temperature of LCAT activity measurement. In addition, Chol distribution between bulk bilayer and boundary layer of PC molecules adjacent to apolipoprotein molecule may influence k_{cat}^{app} . The inclusion of both cholesterol [26;60] and cholesteryl ester [4] molecules into boundary layer in discoidal HDL has been experimentally evidenced.

Finally, the k'_4 value for deletion mutant compared to plasma and wild type apoA-I decreased significantly. The primary importance of the central helices 5, 6 (amino acids in position 143-164) and 7 [16] and mutations clustered in or at the vicinity of helix 4 (residues 146-187) of apoA-I [61], based on the alternative X-ray crystal structure [6] has been suggested earlier. Three arginine residues at positions 149, 153 and 160, with the highest effect of the latter, contribute directly into apoA-I effect on LCAT activity [18]; the significance of R160 has been independently confirmed [15]. It is of importance that all three arginines do not form the interchain salt bridge with negatively charged residues in double superhelix model [12] that locates two apoA-I molecules on the surface of discoidal HDL. However, arginine residues may directly interact with cholesterol molecules [19] and Arg-Chol interaction may determine LCAT catalytic efficiency. In addition, cholesterol accumulation in discoidal HDL induced an abrupt change in conformational stability of two individual domains in apoA-I molecule [24] that may originate from arginine-cholesterol interaction. Arginine has been suggested to induce intrinsic disorder in the structure of exchangeable apolipoproteins [21]. The central helix 6 deleted in Δ139-170 apoA-I may contribute into proper positioning of neighbouring cholesterol molecules relative to Ser181 in LCAT active center, thus switching cholesterol molecule(s) from shielded into "active"-like state with high reactivity [62]. This Chol "activation" by apolipoprotein moiety may be diminished by Chol-complexing phospholipids. Indeed, inhibition of LCAT activity by sphingomyelin has been evidenced [63-65]. The location of R160 at the beginning of flexible solvent-exposed loop in both solar flares [17] and double superhelix [12] models of lipid-bound apoA-I would facilitate multiple hydrogen bonds between the arginine guanidinium group and lipid polar groups. The substrate (PC) activation by apoA-I by increasing the exposure of phosphatidylcholine ester bond to active center of LCAT with the involvement of three arginine residues has been proposed by us recently [24]. This suggestion may be extended now by the inclusion of Arg160 into sequential positioning of substrate and nucleophile molecules in the enzyme active center. The possible involvement of any other residue(s) in helix 6 in apoA-I molecule into LCAT activity remains to be clarified.

The present findings may be related to other apolipoproteins able to activate LCAT. ApoA-I and apoA-IV are the two most efficient cofactors for LCAT [66], apoE and apoC-I still being able to increase the enzyme activity though less efficiently [3], that assumes some difference in LCAT activation by these apolipoproteins. Indeed, LCAT reaction towards discoidal complexes with individual apolipoproteins was characterized by similar but different values [67]. In addition, LCAT activation by apoA-I, apoE and apoC-I was dependent differently on acyl chain saturation [68;69]. LCAT-activating motif in apoA-IV was suggested [66] to include sequence 117-160. Importantly, LCAT-activating motifs in both apoA-I- and apoA-IV structure include single LRT (Leu-Arg-Thr) sequence. ApoE3 molecule contains eight LR* elements throughout the sequence; in addition, apoC-I molecule contains R23 in flexible lipid-binding region of N-domain responsible for LCAT activation [70]. The LR* element exists in the structure of apoC-II - a cofactor of LPL activity that involves also a serine acyl-enzyme intermediate [71]. Oppositely, arginine residues are absent in apoA-II molecule not able to activate LCAT. Thus, it is reasonable to suggest the involvement of LR* element in the influence of apolipoprotein cofactors on (phospho)lipase activities of LCAT and LPL.

Conclusion

The full kinetic analysis of LCAT activity on interface of discoidal HDL with specific apolipoprotein requires the serial measurements of LCAT activity towards particles with varying cholesterol content. An analysis of apparent kinetic parameters at a single Chol concentration together with independently measured dissociation constant for LCAT binding to HDL surface permits to compare the rates of acyl-enzyme formation and its hydrolysis/solvolysis by water and cholesterol. The deletion of 139-170 region in apoA-I structure drastically reduces apolipoprotein ability to activate LCAT by reducing the rate of solvolysis of acyl-enzyme intermediate by cholesterol. This effect is suggested to originate from the proper positioning of phosphatidylcholine ester bond and cholesterol hydroxyl group by arginine residues in this region, in particular R160. The apoA-I-dependent drop in LCAT activity results in RCT impairment that contributes directly into atherosclerosis progression.

The financial support of the Russian Foundation for Basic Research (grant # 10-04-00270) is greatly acknowledged. I thank Dr. M. Rosseneu and Dr. B. Vanloo for providing LCAT and reconstituted discoidal HDL.

References

[1] Frank, P. G. and Marcel, Y. L. (2000). Apolipoprotein A-I: structure-function relationships. *J. Lipid Res.*, *41*, 853-872.

[2] Sorci-Thomas, M. G. and Thomas, M. J. (2002). The effects of altered apolipoprotein A-I structure on plasma HDL concentration. *Trends Cardiovasc. Med.*, *12*, 121-128.

[3] Jonas, A. (2000). Lecithin cholesterol acyltransferase. *Biochim. Biophys. Acta*, *1529*, 245-256.

[4] Dergunov, A. D., Shabrova, E. V. and Dobretsov, G. E. (2010). Composition, structure and substrate properties of reconstituted discoidal HDL with apolipoprotein A-I and cholesteryl ester. *Spectrochim. Acta A Mol. Biomol. Spectrosc.*, *75*, 1100-1107.

[5] Tanaka, M., Koyama, M., Dhanasekaran, P., Nguyen, D., Nickel, M., Lund-Katz, S., Saito, H. and Phillips, M. C. (2008). Influence of tertiary structure domain properties on the functionality of apolipoprotein A-I. *Biochemistry*, *47*, 2172-2180.

[6] Ajees, A. A., Anantharamaiah, G. M., Mishra, V. K., Hussain, M. M. and Murthy, H. M. (2006). Crystal structure of human apolipoprotein A-I: insights into its protective effect against cardiovascular diseases. *Proc. Natl. Acad. Sci. USA.*, *103*, 2126-2131.

[7] Chen, B., Ren, X., Neville, T., Jerome, W. G., Hoyt, D. W., Sparks, D., Ren, G. and Wang, J. (2009). Apolipoprotein AI tertiary structures determine stability and phospholipid-binding activity of discoidal high-density lipoprotein particles of different sizes. *Protein Sci.*, *18*, 921-935.

[8] Chetty, P. S., Mayne, L., Lund-Katz, S., Stranz, D., Englander, S. W. and Phillips, M. C. (2009). Helical structure and stability in human apolipoprotein A-I by hydrogen exchange and mass spectrometry. *Proc. Natl. Acad. Sci. USA.*, *106*, 19005-19010.

[9] Gu, F., Jones, M. K., Chen, J., Patterson, J. C., Catte, A., Jerome, W. G., Li, L. and Segrest, J. P. (2010). Structures of discoidal high density lipoproteins: a combined computational-experimental approach. *J. Biol. Chem.*, *285*, 4652-4665.

[10] Phillips, J. C., Wriggers, W., Li, Z., Jonas, A. and Schulten, K. (1997). Predicting the structure of apolipoprotein A-I in reconstituted high-density lipoprotein disks. *Biophys. J.*, *73*, 2337-2346.

[11] Segrest, J. P., Jones, M. K., Klon, A. E., Sheldahl, C. J., Hellinger, M., De Loof, H. and Harvey, S. C. (1999). A detailed molecular belt model for apolipoprotein A-I in discoidal high density lipoprotein. *J. Biol. Chem.*, *274*, 31755-31758.

[12] Wu, Z., Gogonea, V., Lee, X., Wagner, M. A., Li, X. M., Huang, Y., Undurti, A., May, R. P., Haertlein, M., Moulin, M., Gutsche, I., Zaccai, G., Didonato, J. A. and Hazen, S. L. (2009). Double superhelix model of high density lipoprotein. *J. Biol. Chem.*, *284*, 36605-36619.

[13] Dolphin, P. J. (1992). In M.Rosseneu (ed.), *Structure and Function of Apolipoproteins,* (pp. 295-362). Boca Raton, FL: CRC Press.

[14] Laccotripe, M., Makrides, S. C., Jonas, A. and Zannis, V. I. (1997). The carboxyl-terminal hydrophobic residues of apolipoprotein A-I affect its rate of phospholipid binding and its association with high density lipoprotein. *J. Biol. Chem.*, *272*, 17511-17522.

[15] Cho, K. H., Durbin, D. M. and Jonas, A. (2001). Role of individual amino acids of apolipoprotein A-I in the activation of lecithin:cholesterol acyltransferase and in HDL rearrangements. *J. Lipid Res.*, *42*, 379-389.

[16] Sorci-Thomas, M. G., Bhat, S. and Thomas, M. J. (2009). Activation of lecithin:cholesterol acyltransferase by HDL ApoA-I central helices. *Clin. Lipidol.*, *4*, 113-124.

[17] Wu, Z., Wagner, M. A., Zheng, L., Parks, J. S., Shy, J. M. 3., Smith, J. D., Gogonea, V. and Hazen, S. L. (2007). The refined structure of nascent HDL reveals a key functional domain for particle maturation and dysfunction. *Nat. Struct. Mol. Biol.*, *14*, 861-868.

[18] Roosbeek, S., Vanloo, B., Duverger, N., Caster, H., Breyne, J., De Beun, I., Patel, H., Vandekerckhove, J., Shoulders, C., Rosseneu, M. and Peelman, F. (2001). Three arginine residues in apolipoprotein A-I are critical for activation of lecithin:cholesterol acyltransferase. *J. Lipid Res.*, *42*, 31-40.

[19] Klimov, A. N., Kozhevnikova, K. A., Klueva, N. N. and Belova, E. V. (1992). On the mechanism of cholesterol interaction with apolipoproteins A-I and E. *Chem. Phys. Lipids, 62*, 229-237.

[20] Cheng, Y., LeGall, T., Oldfield, C. J., Dunker, A. K. and Uversky, V. N. (2006). Abundance of intrinsic disorder in protein associated with cardiovascular disease. *Biochemistry, 45*, 10448-10460.

[21] Dergunov, A. D. (2011). Local/bulk determinants of conformational stability of exchangeable apolipoproteins. *Biochim. Biophys. Acta, 1814*, 1169-1177.

[22] Rousset, X., Vaisman, B., Amar, M., Sethi, A. A. and Remaley, A. T. (2009). Lecithin: cholesterol acyltransferase--from biochemistry to role in cardiovascular disease. *Curr. Opin. Endocrinol. Diabetes Obes., 16*, 163-171.

[23] Dergunov, A. D. (2011). Kinetic analysis of lecithin:cholesterol acyltransferase activity toward discoidal HDL. *Lipids, 46*, 1075-1079.

[24] Dergunov, A. D. (2012). A mechanistic model of lecithin:cholesterol acyltransferase activity exploits discoidal HDL composition and structure. *Arch. Biochem. Biophys.*, *520*, 81-87.

[25] Holvoet, P., Zhao, Z., Vanloo, B., Vos, R., Deridder, E., Dhoest, A., Taveirne, J., Brouwers, E., Demarsin, E., Engelborghs, Y., Rosseneu, M., Collen, D. and Brasseur, R. (1995). Phospholipid binding and lecithin-cholesterol acyltransferase activation properties of apolipoprotein A-I mutants. *Biochemistry, 34*, 13334-13342.

[26] Dergunov, A. D., Taveirne, J., Vanloo, B., Caster, H. and Rosseneu, M. (1997). Structural organization of lipid phase and protein-lipid interface in apolipoprotein-phospholipid recombinants: influence of cholesterol. *Biochim. Biophys. Acta, 1346*, 131-146.

[27] Ahmad, S., Gromiha, M. M. and Sarai, A. (2003). RVP-net: online prediction of real valued accessible surface area of proteins from single sequences. *Bioinformatics, 19*, 1849-1851.

[28] Adimoolam, S.andJonas, A. (1997). Identification of a domain of lecithin-cholesterol acyltransferase that is involved in interfacial recognition. *Biochem. Biophys. Res. Comm.*, *232*, 783-787.

[29] Smaby, J. M., Kulkarni, V. S., Momsen, M. and Brown, R. E. (1996). The interfacial elastic packing interactions of galactosylceramides, sphingomyelins, and phosphatidylcholines. *Biophys. J., 70*, 868-877.

[30] Smaby, J. M., Momsen, M. M., Brockman, H. L. and Brown, R. E. (1997). Phosphatidylcholine Acyl Unsaturation Modulates the Decrease in Interfacial Elasticity Induced by Cholesterol. *Biophys J.*, *73*, 1492-1505.

[31] Scott, B. R., McManus, D. C., Franklin, V., McKenzie, A. G., Neville, T., Sparks, D. L. and Marcel, Y. L. (2001). The N-terminal globular domain and the first class A amphipathic helix of apolipoprotein A-I are important for lecithin:cholesterol acyltransferase activation and the maturation of high density lipoprotein in vivo. *J. Biol. Chem.*, *276*, 48716-48724.

[32] Weers, P. M., Patel, A. B., Wan, L. C., Guigard, E., Kay, C. M., Hafiane, A., McPherson, R., Marcel, Y. L. and Kiss, R. S. (2011). Novel N-terminal mutation of human apolipoprotein A-I reduces self-association and impairs LCAT activation. *J. Lipid Res.*, *52*, 35-44.

[33] Chroni, A., Kan, H. Y., Shkodrani, A., Liu, T. and Zannis, V. I. (2005). Deletions of helices 2 and 3 of human apoA-I are associated with severe dyslipidemia following adenovirus-mediated gene transfer in apoA-I-deficient mice. *Biochemistry,* 44, 4108-4117.

[34] Sviridov, D., Hoang, A., Sawyer, W. H. and Fidge, N. H. (2000). Identification of a sequence of apolipoprotein A-I associated with the activation of Lecithin:Cholesterol acyltransferase. *J. Biol. Chem.*, *275*, 19707-19712.

[35] Chroni, A., Duka, A., Kan, H. Y., Liu, T. and Zannis, V. I. (2005). Point mutations in apolipoprotein A-I mimic the phenotype observed in patients with classical lecithin:cholesterol acyltransferase deficiency. *Biochemistry, 44*, 14353-14366.

[36] Chroni, A., Kan, H. Y., Kypreos, K. E., Gorshkova, I. N., Shkodrani, A. and Zannis, V. I. (2004). Substitutions of glutamate 110 and 111 in the middle helix 4 of human apolipoprotein A-I (apoA-I) by alanine affect the structure and in vitro functions of apoA-I and induce severe hypertriglyceridemia in apoA-I-deficient mice. *Biochemistry, 43*, 10442-10457.

[37] Sorci-Thomas, M. G., Curtiss, L., Parks, J. S., Thomas, M. J., Kearns, M. W. and Landrum, M. (1998). The hydrophobic face orientation of apolipoprotein A-I amphipathic helix domain 143-164 regulates lecithin:cholesterol acyltransferase activation. *J. Biol. Chem.*, *273*, 11776-11782.

[38] Dhoest, A., Zhao, Z., De Geest, B., Deridder, E., Sillen, A., Engelborghs, Y., Collen, D. and Holvoet, P. (1997). Role of the Arg123-Tyr166 paired helix of apolipoprotein A-I in lecithin:cholesterol acyltransferase activation. *J. Biol. Chem.*, *272*, 15967-15972.

[39] Daum, U., Langer, C., Duverger, N., Emmanuel, F., Benoit, P., Dene`fle, P., Chirazi, A., Cullen, P., Pritchard, P. H., Bruckert, E., Assmann, G. and von Eckardstein, A. (1999). Apolipoprotein A-I (R151C)Paris is defective in activation of lecithin:cholesterol acyltransferase but not in initial lipid binding, formation of reconstituted lipoproteins, or promotion of cholesterol efflux. *J. Mol. Med. (Berl).*, *77*, 614-622.

[40] Cho, K. H.andJonas, A. (2000). A key point mutation (V156E) affects the structure and functions of human apolipoprotein A-I. *J. Biol. Chem.*, *275*, 26821-26827.

[41] Han, J. M., Jeong, T. S., Lee, W. S., Choi, I. and Cho, K. H. (2005). Structural and functional properties of V156K and A158E mutants of apolipoprotein A-I in the lipid-free and lipid-bound states. *J. Lipid Res., 46*, 589-596.

[42] Daum, U., Leren, T. P., Langer, C., Chirazi, A., Cullen, P., Pritchard, P. H., Assmann, G. and von Eckardstein, A. (1999). Multiple dysfunctions of two apolipoprotein A-I variants, apoA-I(R160L)Oslo and apoA-I(P165R), that are associated with hypoalphalipoproteinemia in heterozygous carriers. *J. Lipid Res.*, *40*, 486-494.

[43] Martín-Campos, J. M., Julve, J., Escolà, J. C., Ordoñez-Llanos, J., Gómez, J., Binimelis, J., González-Sastre, F. and Blanco-Vaca, F. (2002). ApoA-I(MALLORCA) impairs LCAT activation and induces dominant familial hypoalphalipoproteinemia. *J. Lipid Res.*, *43*, 115-123.

[44] Sorci-Thomas, M., Kearns, M. W. and Lee, J. P. (1993). Apolipoprotein A-I domains involved in lecithin-cholesterol acyltransferase activation. Structure:function relationships. *J. Biol. Chem.*, *268*, 21403-21409.

[45] Minnich, A., Collet, X., Roghani, A., Cladaras, C., Hamilton, R. L., Fielding, C. J. and Zannis, V. I. (1992). Site-directed mutagenesis and structure-function analysis of the human apolipoprotein A-I. Relation between lecithin-cholesterol acyltransferase activation and lipid binding. *J. Biol. Chem.*, *267*, 16553-16560.

[46] Rall, S. C. Jr., Weisgraber, K. H., Mahley, R. W., Ogawa, Y., Fielding, C. J., Utermann, G., Haas, J., Steinmetz, A., Menzel, H. J. and Assmann, G. (1984). Abnormal lecithin:cholesterol acyltransferase activation by a human apolipoprotein A-I variant in which a single lysine residue is deleted. *J. Biol. Chem.*, *259*, 10063-10070.

[47] Tilly-Kiesi, M., Zhang, Q., Ehnholm, S., Kahri, J., Lahdenpera", S., Ehnholm, C. and Taskinen, M. R. (1995). ApoA-IHelsinki (Lys107-->0) associated with reduced HDL cholesterol and LpA-I:A-II deficiency. *Arterioscler. Thromb. Vasc. Biol.*, *15*, 1294-1306.

[48] Utermann, G., Haas, J., Steinmetz, A., Paetzold, R., Rall, S. C. Jr., Weisgraber, K. H. and Mahley, R. W. (1984). Apolipoprotein A-IGiessen (Pro143----Arg). A mutant that is defective in activating lecithin:cholesterol acyltransferase. *Eur. J. Biochem.*, *144*, 325-331.

[49] Miettinen, H. E., Jauhiainen, M., Gylling, H., Ehnholm, S., Paloma"ki, A., Miettinen, T. A. and Kontula, K. (1997). Apolipoprotein A-IFIN (Leu159-->Arg) mutation affects lecithin cholesterol acyltransferase activation and subclass distribution of HDL but not cholesterol efflux from fibroblasts. *Arterioscler. Thromb. Vasc. Biol.*, *17*, 3021-3032.

[50] McManus, D. C., Scott, B. R., Frank, P. G., Franklin, V., Schultz, J. R. and Marcel, Y. L. (2000). Distinct central amphipathic alpha-helices in apolipoprotein A-I contribute to the in vivo maturation of high density lipoprotein by either activating lecithin-cholesterol acyltransferase or binding lipids. *J. Biol. Chem.*, *275*, 5043-5051.

[51] Miccoli, R., Zhu, Y., Daum, U., Wessling, J., Huang, Y., Navalesi, R., Assmann, G. and von Eckardstein, A. (1997). A natural apolipoprotein A-I variant, apoA-I (L141R)Pisa, interferes with the formation of alpha-high density lipoproteins (HDL) but not with the formation of pre beta 1-HDL and influences efflux of cholesterol into plasma. *J. Lipid Res.*, *38*, 1242-1253.

[52] Recalde, D., Velez-Carrasco, W., Civeira, F., Cenarro, A., Gomez-Coronado, D., Ordovas, J. M. and Pocovi, M. (2001). Enhanced fractional catabolic rate of apo A-I and apo A-II in heterozygous subjects for apo A-I(Zaragoza) (L144R). *Atherosclerosis, 154*, 613-623.

[53] Huang, W., Sasaki, J., Matsunaga, A., Nanimatsu, H., Moriyama, K., Han, H., Kugi, M., Koga, T., Yamaguchi, K. and Arakawa, K. (1998). A novel homozygous missense mutation in the apo A-I gene with apo A-I deficiency. *Arterioscler. Thromb. Vasc. Biol.*, *18*, 389-396.

[54] Miller, M., Aiello, D., Pritchard, H., Friel, G. and Zeller, K. (1998). Apolipoprotein A-I(Zavalla) (Leu159-->Pro): HDL cholesterol deficiency in a kindred associated with premature coronary artery disease. *Arterioscler. Thromb. Vasc. Biol.*, *18*, 1242-1247.

[55] Moriyama, K., Sasaki, J., Takada, Y., Matsunaga, A., Fukui, J., Albers, J. J. and Arakawa, K. (1996). A cysteine-containing truncated apo A-I variant associated with HDL deficiency. *Arterioscler. Thromb. Vasc. Biol.*, *16*, 1416-1423.
[56] Funke, H., von Eckardstein, A., Pritchard, P. H., Karas, M., Albers, J. J. and Assmann, G. (1991). A frameshift mutation in the human apolipoprotein A-I gene causes high density lipoprotein deficiency, partial lecithin: cholesterol-acyltransferase deficiency, and corneal opacities. *J. Clin. Invest.*, *87*, 371-376.
[57] Bolin, D. J.andJonas, A. (1994). Binding of lecithin:cholesterol acyltransferase to reconstituted high density lipoproteins is affected by their lipid but not apolipoprotein composition. *J. Biol. Chem.*, *269*, 7429-7434.
[58] Miller, K. R.andParks, J. S. (1997). Influence of vesicle surface composition on the interfacial binding of lecithin:cholesterol acyltransferase and apolipoprotein A-I. *J. Lipid Res.*, *38*, 1094-1102.
[59] Parks, J. S., Huggins, K. W., Gebre, A. K. and Burleson, E. R. (2000). Phosphatidylcholine fluidity and structure affect lecithin:cholesterol acyltransferase activity. *J. Lipid Res.*, *41*, 546-553.
[60] Dergunov, A. D., Dobretsov, G. E., Visvikis, S. and Siest, G. (2001). Protein-lipid interactions in reconstituted high density lipoproteins: apolipoprotein and cholesterol influence. *Chem. Phys. Lipids, 113*, 67-82.
[61] Koukos, G., Chroni, A., Duka, A., Kardassis, D. and Zannis, V. I. (2007). Naturally occurring and bioengineered apoA-I mutations that inhibit the conversion of discoidal to spherical HDL: the abnormal HDL phenotypes can be corrected by treatment with LCAT. *Biochem. J.*, *406*, 167-174.
[62] Lange, Y.andSteck, T. L. (2008). Cholesterol homeostasis and the escape tendency (activity) of plasma membrane cholesterol. *Prog. Lipid Res.*, *47*, 319-332.
[63] Bolin, D. J.andJonas, A. (1996). Sphingomyelin inhibits the lecithin-cholesterol acyltransferase reaction with reconstituted high density lipoproteins by decreasing enzyme binding. *J. Biol. Chem, 271*, 19152-19158.
[64] Sparks, D. L., Frank, P. G. and Neville, T. A. (1998). Effect of the surface lipid composition of reconstituted LPA-I on apolipoprotein A-I structure and lecithin: cholesterol acyltransferase activity. *Biochim. Biophys. Acta, 1390*, 160-172.
[65] Subbaiah, P. V., Horvath, P. and Achar, S. B. (2006). Regulation of the activity and fatty acid specificity of lecithin-cholesterol acyltransferase by sphingomyelin and its metabolites, ceramide and ceramide phosphate. *Biochemistry, 45*, 5029-5038.
[66] Emmanuel, F., Steinmetz, A., Rosseneu, M., Brasseur, R., Gosselet, N., Attenot, F., Cuine, S., Seguret, S., Latta, M. and Fruchart, J. C. (1994). Identification of specific amphipathic alpha-helical sequence of human apolipoprotein A-IV involved in lecithin:cholesterol acyltransferase activation. *J. Biol. Chem, 269*, 29883-29890.
[67] Jonas, A., Sweeny, S. A. and Herbert, P. N. (1984). Discoidal complexes of A and C apolipoproteins with lipids and their reactions with lecithin: cholesterol acyltransferase. *J. Biol. Chem.*, *259*, 6369-6375.

[68] Soutar, A. K., Garner, C. W., Baker, H. N., Sparrow, J. T., Jackson, R. L., Gotto, A. M. and Smith, L. C. (1975). Effect of the human plasma apolipoproteins and phosphatidylcholine acyl donor on the activity of lecithin: cholesterol acyltransferase. *Biochemistry, 14*, 3057-3064.

[69] Steinmetz, A., Kaffarnik, H. and Utermann, G. (1985). Activation of phosphatidylcholine-sterol acyltransferase by human apolipoprotein E isoforms. *Eur. J. Biochem., 152*, 747-751.

[70] James, P. F., Dogovski, C., Dobson, R. C., Bailey, M. F., Goldie, K. N., Karas, J. A., Scanlon, D. B., O'Hair, R. A. and Perugini, M. A. (2009). Aromatic residues in the C-terminal helix of human apoC-I mediate phospholipid interactions and particle morphology. *J. Lipid Res., 50*, 1384-1394.

[71] Rojas, C., Wang, H. H., Lively, C. R., Gustafson, W. G., Schulz, L. O. and McFarland, J. T. (1989). Spectral observation of an acyl-enzyme intermediate of lipoprotein lipase. *Biochemistry, 28,* 4475-4481.

In: Apolipoproteins
Editors: A. D. Sidorov and M. Y. Nikitin
ISBN: 978-1-62257-484-1

Chapter VII

Regulation by FGF-1 of apoE/HDL Generation in Astrocytes

Jinichi Ito* and Makoto Michikawa
Biochemistry, Graduate School of Medical Sciences, Nagoya City University,
Kawasumi 1, Mizuho-cho, Mizuho-ku, Nagoya, Japan

Abstract

The neural cells in the central nervous system (CNS) are segregated by the blood-brain barrier (BBB) from cholesterol transporters such as low density lipoproteins (LDL) and very low density lipoproteins (VLDL) in human blood plasma, although the CNS is an organ to require cholesterol at very high level. Therefore, cholesterol homeostasis in the CNS is surely controlled by the brain-specific cholesterol transport system. Apolipoprotein E (apoE) produced by astrocytes is a most abundant apolipoprotein in the cerebrospinal fluid (CSF). Astrocytes generate cholesterol-rich high density lipoprotein (apoE/HDL) by using the endogenous apoE and phospholipid-rich and cholesterol-poor HDL (apoA-I/HDL) through the interaction with exogenous apoA-I which is probably produced by brain endothelial cells.

The secretion of endogenous apoE from rat astrocytes is started within 30 min after the initiation of biosynthesis. The apoE secreted from rat astrocytes uses pre-synthesized cholesterol rather than newly-synthesized cholesterol for biogenesis of HDL, although exogenous human apoE mediates effluxes of both pre-synthesized and newly synthesized cholesterols as well as exogenous cyclodextrin. This suggests that astrocytes secrete hardly endogenous apoE as a lipid-free apoE.

Rat astrocytes cultured for one month (long-term cultured astrocytes) enhance significantly generation of apoE/HDL dependently on fibroblast growth factor 1 (FGF-1) produced by astrocytes in the manner of apparent autocrine action. The release of FGF-1 is likely provoked by oxidative stress involved in long-term cultured stress. Purified FGF-1 enhances the apoE/HDL generation of astrocytes accompanied with enhancing syntheses of both apoE and cholesterol. FGF-1 increases cholesterol synthesis through the activation of MAP kinase cascade in astrocytes, stimulates intracellular apoE

*E-mail: jitoh@med.nagoya-cu.ac.jp.

transport through PI3-kinase/Akt pathway and enhances apoE mRNA expression through increasing mRNA expression of LXRα.

The mechanism underlying FGF-1 release from astrocytes and subsequent generation of apoE/HDL are important issues to be addressed to understand the role of FGF-1 in damaged brains, including bran injury, brain inflammation, or neurodegenerative diseases. The regulation by FGF-1 of apoE/HDL generation under the stress-conditions is mainly argued on the base of our experimental results including recently obtained and unpublished several data in this chapter.

Introduction

Cholesterol is an important component lipid of cell membrane. The hydroxyl group of cholesterol molecule is located near the hydrophilic head of phospholipid molecule and the flat steroid structure is filled up among hydrocarbon chains of phospholipids molecules. Such a feature of chemical structure in cholesterol molecule is useful for regulation of fluidity and viscosity of cell membrane. Cholesterol, furthermore, has a high affinity for sphingomyelin and constructs a membrane lipid raft, a cholesterol- and sphingomyelin-rich domain, to offer a platform for molecules participating in signal transductions in the plasma membrane.

The CNS requires highly cholesterol, because neural cells such as neurons, astrocytes, oligodendroglias and microglias own complicated morphology with huge amount of plasma membrane and oligodendroglias organize myelin structure. Indeed, the CNS is a cholesterol-rich organ, in which approximately 20 - 25 % of total body cholesterol is localized to maintain functions and viability of neural cells [1]. The BBB, however, segregates neurons and glias in the brain from the systemic circulation and a major lipid transporter in human blood plasma, such as LDL. Therefore there is a unique and specific system for cholesterol delivery to neural cells to maintain cholesterol homeostasis in the brain. Lipoporteins found in the CSF are all HDL but not LDL or VLDL. Apolipoproteins identified in HDL of the CSF are mainly apoE and apoA-I in addition to minor apolipoproteins such as apolipoproteins A-IV, D and J [4,30]. The apoE produced and secreted by astrocytes functions dominantly in intercellular cholesterol transport between neural cells in the brain. The apoE appears to be un-exchangeable with the plasma apoE, because the phenotype of apoE in the CNS of recipient remains unchanged even after liver transplantation [36]. Therefore, the intercellular cholesterol transport in CNS is thought to be mediated by the HDL generated within the brain.

FGF-1 (acidic FGF, heparin- binding growth factor 1, HBGF-1) is one of members of FGF family and stimulates proliferation and differentiation of mesodermal and neuroectodermal cells as well as FGF-2 (basic FGF) [8,33]. FGF-1 isolated from neural tissue as a Mr 16,000 – 18,000 polypeptide is 55% identical in amino acid sequence with FGF-2. Many kinds of cell species produce and release FGF-1 in addition to FGF-2 at low level. In the brain, both FGF-1 and FGF-2 are distributed exhibiting the different localization. FGF-1 is known to be localized in all motor neurons and primary sensory neurons in the mesencephalon and much less in a small number of glial cells of white matter [9,10]. FGF-2 is mainly expressed in astrocytes and pyramidal neurons of the hippocampus [9]. FGF-1 appears to contribute to neuron survival and neurite outgrowth in vitro and in vivo [18,49]. In

Alzheimer brains, astrocytes are stained for FGF-1 more strongly than those in control brains in both gray and white matters [52].

FGF-1 binds with all receptor isoforms such as FGF receptor 1 (FGFR1), FGFR2, FGFR3 and FGFR4 [47]. FGF-1 is likely synthesized and localized in the cytosol and nucleus of the producing cells, because it has no amino-terminal signal sequence for secretion as well as FGF-2 [39,57]. There is a report that disruption of endoplasmic reticulum (ER)-Golgi communication by brefeldin A has no effect on FGF-1 release from the producing cells [5], suggesting that the FGF-1 release to extracellular space is unlikely to be mediated by the classical intracellular transport system through the ER/Golgi pathway after the biosynthesis. The mechanism of FGF-1 release is unclear at present in spite of many previous investigations. We found that astrocytes enhance the production and release of FGF-under (acidic FGF, heparin-binding growth factor 1, HBGF-1) stressful condition such as long-term culture and cryoinjury [23,44,49,53]. FGF-1 enhances apoE/HDL generation of astrocytes accompanied by the up-regulation of syntheses of apoE and cholesterol in the autocrine or paracrine manner [24,44].

1. HDL Generation Mediated by Endogenous apoE and Exogenous apoA-I in Astrocytes

Human apoE composed of 299 amino acid residues is a glycoprotein with molecular weight of 37 kDa. ApoE is produced and secreted by many kinds of cells such as macrophages, steroid-producing cells, liver and small intestine in the peripheral tissues. In the CNS, apoE is mainly produced by astrocytes and partly by microglias [12]. The production of apoE is enhanced accompanied with brain development or regeneration of injured neurons [48]. Astrocytes secreted apoE along with cellular cholesterol and phospholipids as apoE/HDL particles with 10 – 17 nm in diameter. Astrocytes secrete apoJ also as smaller HDL (7.5 – 12 nm in diameter).

The mechanism of apoE secretion from astrocytes is unclear at present. We studied the mechanism of apoE secretion by using astrocytes prepared from fetal rat brain. Here, we describe regarding the mechanism for apoE secretion and apoE/HDL generation in astrocytes on the base of unpublished recent our data. The secretion of ^{35}S-labeled apoE started within 30 min in rat astrocytes. At 10 min after the start of metabolic biosynthesis of apoE with ^{35}S-methionine, ^{35}S-apoE was collected from the intracellular membrane fraction containing mainly lipid raft domain, suggesting that the intracellular apoE associates with lipid raft in the inside of Golgi apparatus or endosome in the process of intracellular transport of apoE. The apoE was secreted from wild-type mouse as apoE/HDL particles with density of 1.08 – 1.12 g/mL, while the astrocytes prepared from ATP-binding cassette transporter A1-deficient (ABCA1-KO) mouse secreted apoE as insufficiently lipidated HDL with higher density (d = 1.12 – 1.17 g/mL) into the conditioned medium. The intracellular apoE in ABCA1-KO astrocytes was collected from the non-lipid raft with higher density unlike that in wild type astrocytes (unpublished data), suggesting that ABCA1 is necessary to translocate apoE onto lipid raft for generation of mature HDL. This result has been confirmed by the different culture system using rat astrocytoma GA-1 cells, which express very low level of mRNAs of apoE and ABCA1 [22]. In rat apoE-transfected GA-1 cells (GA-1/25), the secreted apoE was recovered with the HDL fractions with higher density similarly to the apoE secreted from ABCA1-KO astrocytes. When GA-1/25 cells were treated with TO901317, a LXR agonist, the cellular level of ABCA1 was increased in GA-1/25 cells. The intracellular apoE, furthermore, was increased in the membrane lipid raft fraction along with ABCA1 and the secreted apoE was collected from the apoE-HDL fraction with lower density as mature apoE/HDL. TO901317 failed to translocate ABCA1 to the lipid raft in GA-1/Mock cells without apoE, although the cellular ABCA1 level was increased in the non-raft domain but not the lipid raft by TO901317. This suggests that high lipidation of apoE for mature apoE/HDL generation is dependent on the enhancement of cellular ABCA1 level and the interaction between apoE and ABCA1 in the lipid raft domain. The membrane-associated apoE, indeed, was precipitated by an anti-ABCA1 antibody through ABCA1, and ABCA1 was also done by using an anti-apoE antibody, even after the cell surface ABCA1 and apoE were digested by the treatment with exogenously added trypsin. Although ABCA1 is generally thought to be distributed in non-lipid raft fraction, the astrocyte's ABCA1 appears to be localized in membrane lipid raft through the interaction with endogenous apoE.

Exogenously added human apoE generates apoE/HDL using both newly synthesized and pre-synthesized cholesterol through the interaction with the cell surface of astrocytes. Surprisingly, the endogenous apoE secreted from rat astrocytes used pre-synthesized cholesterol rather than newly synthesized one for apoE/HDL generation. This implies that the endogenous apoE in astrocytes exports preferentially the pre-synthesized cellular cholesterol to the conditioned medium. If apoE is secreted by astrocytes as a lipid-free apolipoprotein, the endogenous apoE must transport both newly synthesized and presynthesized cholesterol to the extracellular space like exogenously added apoE. Whether the apoE secreted from astrocytes is lipidated in intracellular site is very important issue to be addressed.

The mechanism for apoE secretion has been investigated mainly by using macrophages. After the biosynthesis in the endoplasmic reticulum, some of apoE molecules are likely secreted from the plasma membrane through O-linked glycosylation in the Golgi, while other large parts of apoE are digested in the lysosome [58]. In macrophages, the secreted apoE is re-internalized for the generation of apoE-HDL [59]. ApoE appears to be secreted from macrophages to rely on the functions of protein kinase A and microtubules via calcium-dependent pathway [31]. ABCA1 must participate greatly in apoE secretion, as deficiency of ABCA1 causes the decrease of apoE secretion [17,56].

On the other hand, apoA-I is reportedly produced by brain capillary endothelial cells [42]. Exogenous apoA-I generates phospholipids-rich and cholesterol-poor HDL through the interaction with ABCA1 in the non-lipid raft fraction of astrocytes as well as many kinds of peripheral cells and unlike the case of endogenous apoE in astrocytes [22]. We found a cytosolic lipid-protein particle (CLPP), defined as a lipid-protein complex with density of 1.09 - 1.16 g/ml and diameter 17 - 18 nm like plasma HDL in the cytosol fraction of rat astrocytes [21,25]. The CLPP participates in the intracellular cholesterol trafficking in association with apoA-I-mediated HDL generation. Caveolin-1, protein kinase Cα and cyclophilin A are recovered in the CLPP fraction after the stimulation of astrocytes with apoA-I [19,20]. The apoA-I-mediated cholesterol release is inhibited by cyclosporin A, an inhibitor of cyclophilin A. ApoA-I induces the tyrosine phosphorylation of phospholipase Cγ (PL-Cγ), followed by the translocation of PL-Cγ to the CLPP fraction and diacylglyceride production in the CLPP. The translocation and activation of protein kinase Cα to/in the CLPP are continuously enhanced [29]. The suppression of either phospholipase C or protein kinase C inhibits apoA-I-mediated cholesterol release and apoA-I/HDL generation. These results suggest that the CLPP is an intracellular site of apoA-I-induced signal transduction and has a role as an intracellular cholesterol transporter. The different type of lipoproteins generated by apoE and apo A-I may exhibit different function in the brain [26].

2. Regulation by FGF-1 of apoE/HDL Generation

It is an interesting issue whether the apoE/HDL generation by astrocytes is regulated dependently on cellular cholesterol level of astrocytes or controlled by the unknown system to detect cholesterol level in the brain. We found that some trophic factor is one of regulators for apoE/HDL generation under the stressful conditions. Rat astrocytes enhance syntheses of cholesterol and apoE, resulted in increasing generation of apoE/HDL during long-term culture [23]. The mRNA expression and production of FGF-1 are also increased in rat astrocytes cultured over three weeks. FGF-1 enhances biosyntheses of apoE and cholesterol by an autocrine or paracrine fashion, leading to an enhanced generation of apoE/HDL.

The cholesterol synthesis was enhanced through the phosphorylations of MEK and ERK in rat astrocytes stimulated with FGF-1, implying the dependency of cholesterol synthesis on activation of MAP kinase cascade [24]. In apoE-deficient (apoE-KO) mouse astrocytes, FGF-1 stimulates cholesterol biosynthesis without enhancing its release, indicating a pathway independent of apoE secretion [24]. LY294002, an inhibitor of phosphatidylinositide 3-OH kinase (PI3K), suppressed not only Akt phosphorylation but also apoE secretion and apoE/HDL generation without suppression of cholesterol biosynthesis.

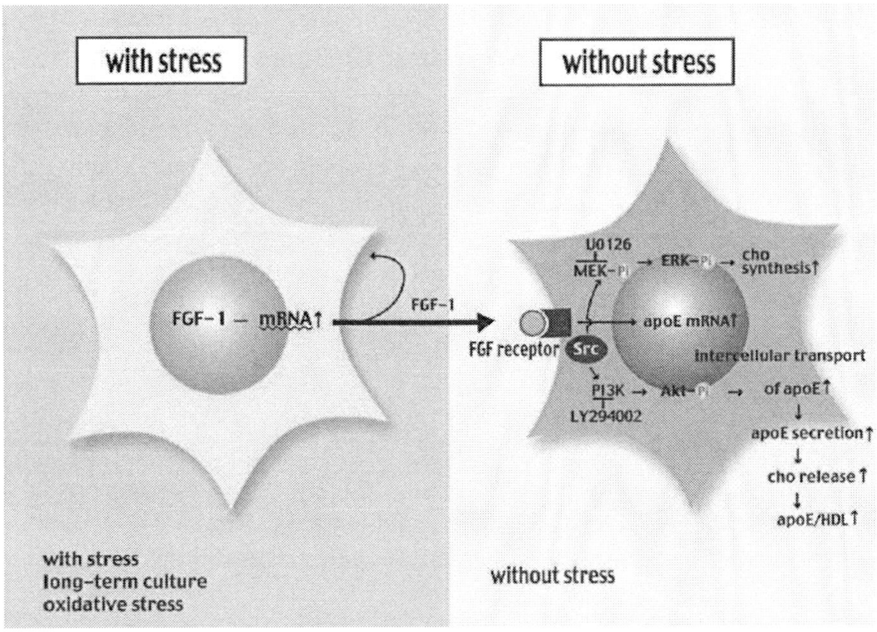

Figure 1. Mechanism of apoE/HDL generation by FGF-1 in rat astrocytes.

This cell signaling and apoE/HDL generation mediated by FGF-1 were suppressed by the inhibition of Src activity [46]. The increase by FGF-1 of apoE mRNA expression is not influenced by either LY294002 or U0126, a MEK inhibitor, in rat astrocytes. Interestingly, the apoE secretion from GA-1/25 cells was increased by FGF-1 and reversed by LY294002, despite of the lack of effect of FGF-1 and LY294002 on the apoE transcription step. As the change of apoE level in the medium and cell is reciprocal, the effect of FGF-1 seems to be on the process of apoE transport/secretion through the activation of PI3K rather than its translation.

FGF-1 increases mRNA expression of liver X receptor α (LXRα) in addition to apoE in rat astrocytes. Increase of LXRα is suppressed by inhibition of the FGF receptor-1 and MEK/ERK but not by inhibition of PI3K/Akt [37]. The liver X receptor element responsible for activation of the rat apoE promoter by FGF-1 is located between -450 and -320bp, and the direct repeat 4 (DR4) element in this region (-448 to -433bp) is responsible for the activation. It was demonstrated by Chromatin immunoprecipitation analysis that FGF-1 enhances association of LXR with the rat apoE promoter. FGF-1 also enhances biosynthesis of LXR ligand, such as 25-hydroxycholesterol. Thus, FGF-1 enhances apoE/HDL generation through at least three different signal transductions in astrocytes (Figure 1).

3. FGF-1 Release from Astrocytes

Rat astrocytes increase the production and release of FGF-1 to enhance apoE/HDL generation under the long-term culture stress and cryo-injury, suggesting that FGF-1 functions as a regulator of apoE/HDL production to contribute to recovery of the brain from damage. We therefore attempted to search a trigger to induce the synthesis and release of FGF-1 in astrocytes under stress conditions to understand regulation system of apoE/HDL generation in the brain. Oxidative stress is one of the common events in the case of brain damage. The release of FGF-1 was enhanced along with cytosolic proteins such as HSP70, HSP90, PK-Cδ and β–actin from both conventional and long-term cultured rat astrocytes by the treatment with 100 μM H_2O_2 without inducing apoptosis in the cells. Hydrogen peroxide, furthermore, increased the permeation of membrane-nonpermeable molecules such as Rhodamine-phalloidin and trypsin into rat astrocytes. The release of [^{35}S]-labeled cytosolic proteins with a wide range of molecular weight was increased by the treatment with H_2O_2 from rat astrocytes, after metabolical labeling with [^{35}S]-methionine. These findings suggest that the release of FGF-1 from astrocytes treated with H_2O_2 is hardly mediated by the mechanism specific to FGF-1 molecule. The hydrogen peroxide-mediated release of cytosolic proteins is suppressed by the treatment with antioxidants. As FGF-1 has no biochemical activity to rat astrocytes damaged with H_2O_2, the FGF-1 released from H_2O_2–treated astrocytes is thought to act much more on healthy astrocytes without stress or injury in the manner of paracrine than on damaged astrocytes in autocrine action. The healthy astrocytes stimulated with FGF-1 are able to produce actively apoE/HDL through the enhancement of biosyntheses and release of apoE and cholesterol. Astrocytes are more sensitive to H_2O_2 than cell lines such as bovine endothelial cells and HepG2 cells for release of cytosolic proteins. Higher sensitivity of astrocytes to oxidative stress may be effective to protect the brain against oxidative stress by using the released FGF-1.

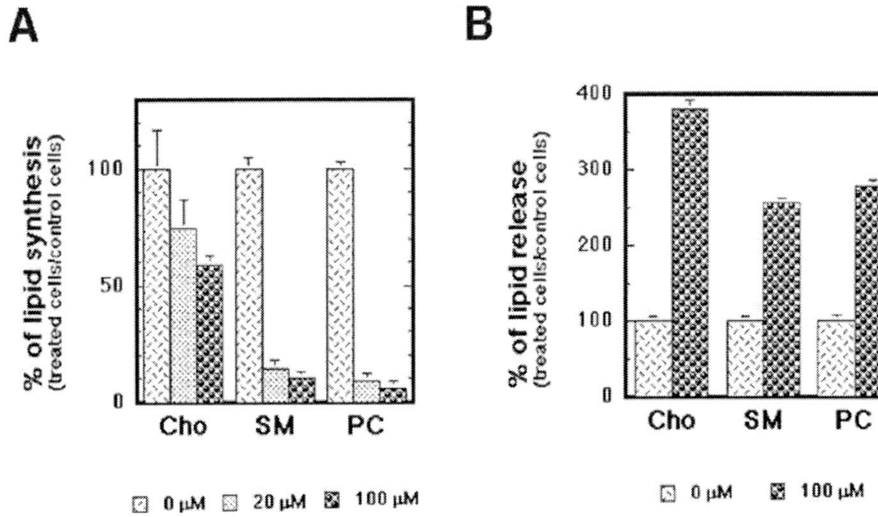

Figure 2. Effects of H2O2 on lipid synthesis and relese in rat astrocytes.

Hydrogen peroxide suppresses transiently biosyntheses of lipids such as cholesterol, phosphatidylcholine and sphingomyelin and enhances lipid release in/from astrocytes (Figure 2). This imply that oxidative stress lowers membrane lipid content of astrocytes by suppression of lipid synthesis and increase in lipid release, makes the membrane unstable and increases membrane-permeability for the release of FGF-1 along with cytosolic proteins. Interestingly, the lipid synthesis of HepG2 and endothelial cells is suppressed by H_2O_2 much less than that of astrocytes. Such findings lead us to the speculation that the sensitive reactivity to oxidative stress for FGF-1 release may be one of important functions of astrocytes to protect the brain against oxidative stress. FGF-1 appears to be localized in the neural tissue as a high molecular weight complex. The complex contains FGF-1 and p40 extravasecular domain of synaptotagmin (Syn)-1, and the brain-derived FGF-1/p40 Syn-1 complex is found associated with the calcium-binding protein, S100A13 [2,34]. FGF-1 is released as a latent homodimer with the p40 extravasecular domain of synaptotagmin (Syn)-1 by heat-shock stress. These reports exhibit that FGF-1 is released as complex forms under the stress conditions, though the biochemical significance of FGF-1/synaptotagmin-1 complex is unclear for FGF-1 release at present.

4. Brain Protection from Injury and Stress by FGF-1 and apoE/HDL

There have been abundantly reported that the apoE/HDL produced by astrocytes participates in development of the CNS to promote synaptogenesis, neurite outgrowth and axon growth [6,11]. ApoE production is dramatically increased in the brain after injury of the rat sciatic and optic nerves [48]. Nerve injury has been observed to stimulate the secretion of apoE by glial cells. With respect to the role(s) of apoE/HDL in the brain injury, apoE reportedly protects against oxidative stress by reducing glutamate toxicity [35]. H. Hayashi et al. reported that apoE/HDL protects neurons from apoptosis through activation of phospholipase Cγ1 and inhibition of calcineurin mediated by LDL receptor-related protein-1 [14,15]. These lines of evidence suggest that the apoE/HDL derived from astrocytes contributes to maintain viability and function of neurons, and protect neuronal cells from stress and injury in the CNS. Thus, why and how apoE/HDL production is enhanced by injury of the brain would be a critical question to be addressed.

It has been well known that FGF-1 is released in response to sublethal cell injury such as oxidative stress, heat shock, hypoxia and serum starvation. The production of FGF-1 has been demonstrated immunohistochemically in the post-injury reactive astrocytes of mice in vivo [45]. FGF-1 is highly expressed in motor neurons and released in response to oxidative stress [3]. Even NIH 3T3 cells transfected with a synthetic gene encoding FGF-1, secrete FGF-1 into the conditioned medium when these cells are exposed to heat shock (at 42 °C for 2 h), but not under the regular conditions at 37 °C [27]. FGF-1 is apparently produced and released in/from astrocytes in response to exposure to stress and injury in the brain. We demonstrated that the productions of FGF-1 and apoE are increased in the astrocytes around the lesion of cryo-injury in the mouse brain [49]. The FGF-1 production was ahead of the increase of apoE synthesis and the wound healing was substantially delayed in the apoE-deficient mice. The production of FGF-1 was obviously increased in the injured brain of apoE-deficient mouse also. These findings imply that cryo-injury promotes astrocytes to produce and secrete FGF-1, which up-regulates the apoE/HDL generation to assists wound healing. In neurodegenerative diseases including Alzheimer's disease, it is known that there is ongoing neuronal damage, inflammation, or generation of oxidative stress, implaying that FGF-1 release may be enhanced in the brain of patients with AD [52]. On the base of these findings, it may be possible to postulate that stress and injury enhance FGF-1 release from astrocytes and the released FGF-1 acts on the healthy astrocytes in the manner of paracrine action to increase the production of apoE/HDL for protection and recovery of neural cells from stress and injury in the brain.

5. Production and Function of FGF-1 and apoE/lipoproteins in Alzheimar's Desease

Because production of FGF-1 is enhanced by the injury or oxidative stress, it is reasonable to assume that its expression level is upregulated in neurodegenerative diseases including Alzheimer disease (AD). It has been reported that FGF-1 expression level is increased in reactive astrocytes surrounding senile plaques and the distribution pattern of FGF-1 receptor shows a similar to that of FGF-1 [50]. FGF-1 expression level in entorhinal cortex is likely decreased in AD brains compared with control cases, while remaining neurons showed significantly higher at FGF-1 immnoreactivity [51], suggesting that not only astrocytes, but also neurons express FGF-1 to protect themselves in the brain. In addition to expression of FGF-1 in human brains, it has been shown that the levels of FGF-1 in the CSF and serum from the patients with AD was significantly higher than in patients without AD [38]. Taken all these results together, it may be possible that in the surrounding area of damaged brain region caused by Aβ deposition in AD brain, astrocytes and some types of neurons enhance synthesis and release of FGF-1, which up-regulates syntheses of apoE and cholesterol leading to enhance generation of apoE/HDL for neuronal repair and protection.

With respect to roles of apoE or cholesterol in AD pathogenesis, it has been reported that cholesterol level in the CSF of patients with AD is decreased compared with those with non-AD disease [7,43]. The major part of cholesterol in the CSF exists as a component of HDL, which is generated by apoE derived from astrocytes in an apoE-isoform-dependent manner [13,40,41]. The generation of HDL by apoE3 is greater than apoE4. Because ABCA1 is a key molecule for apoE-mediated HDL generation to maintain adequate cholesterol homeostasis and distribution, ABCA1 has gained attention as being an important protein target for both AD pathogenesis and treatment.

There are several studies showing that ABCA1 deletion leads to an increase in both amyloid β (Aβ) and amyloid burden in the brains of transgenic mouse models [16,32,54], although ABCA1 deletion did not alter Aβ production [54]. It has been demonstrated that the fully lipidated apoE/HDL was required for Aβ degradation in microglia, indicating that the presence of ABCA1 and subsequent formation of apoE/HDL have an effect on Aβ clearance [28]. The effect of ABCA1 and HDL generation on Aβ clearance has been confirmed by a study using ABCA1 transgenic mice, showing that there was a dramatic decrease in the amount of Aβ deposition [55]. Based on these data, it is possible that the regulation of apoE/HDL level via ABCA1 may be targets for development AD therapies. In addition, because FGF-1 is known to stimulate synthesis of apoE, cholesterol, and phospholipids, leading to increased generation of apoE/HDL, modulation of FGF-1 may be an alterative target for AD therapy.

References

[1] Bjorkhem, i. and Meaney, S., Brain cholesterol: long secret life behind a barrier, *Arterioscler. Thromb. Vasc. Biol.*, 24 (2004) 806-815.

[2] Carreira, C.M., LaVallee, T.M., Tarantini, F., Jackson, A., Lathrop, J.T., Hampton, B., Burgess, W.H. and Maciag, T., S100A13 is involved in the regulation of fibroblast growth factor-1 and P40 synaptotagmin-1 release in vitro, *J. Biol. Chem.*, 273 (1998) 22224-22231.

[3] Cassiana, P., peher, M., Vargas, M.R., Castellanos, R., Barbeito, A.G., Estevez, A.G., Thompson, J.A. and Beckman, J.S., Astrocyte activation by fibroblast growth factor-1 and motor neuron apoptosis: implications for amyotrophic lateral sclerosis, *J. Neurochem.*, 93 (2005) 38-46.

[4] Chiba, H., Mitamura, T., Fujisawa, S.-i., Ogata, A., Aimoto, Y., Tashiro, K. and Kobayashi, K., Apolipoproteins in rat cerebrospinal fluid: a comparison with plasma lipoprotein metabolism and effect of aging, *Neurosci. Letters*, 133 (1991) 207-210.

[5] Christofori, G. and Luef, S., Novel forms od acidic fibroblast growth factor-1are constitutively exported by beta tumor cell lines independent from conventional secretion and apoptosis, *angiogenesis*, 1 (1997) 55-70.

[6] DeMattos, R.B., Curtiss, L.K. and L., W.D., A minimally lipidated form of cell-derived apolipoprotein E exhibits isoform-specific stimulation of neurite outgrowth in the absence of exogenous lipids or lipoproteins, *J. Biol. Chem.*, 273 (1998) 4206-4212.

[7] Demeester, N., Castro, G., Desrumaux, C., De Geitere, C., Fruchart, J.-C., santens, P., Mulleners, E., Engelborghs, S., De Deyn, P.P. and Vandekerckhove, J.,

Characterization and functional studies of lipoproteins, lipid transfer proteins, and lecithin:cholesterol acyltransferase in CSF of normal individuals and patients with Alzheimer's disease, *L. Lipid res.*, 41 (200) 963-974.

[8] Dono, R., Fibloblast growth factors as regulators of central nervous system development and function, *Am. J. Physiol. Regul. Integr. Comp. Physiol.*, 284 (2003) R876-R881.

[9] Eckenstein, F.P., Andersson, C., Kuzis, K. and Woodward, W.G., Distribution of acidic and basic fibroblast growth factors in the mature, injured and developing rat nervous sysem, *Progress Brain Res.*, 103 (1994) 55-63.

[10] Exkenstien, F.P., Fibloblast growth factors in the nervous system, *J. Neurobiol.*, 25 (1994) 1467-1480.

[11] Fagan, A.M., Bu, G., Sun, Y., Daugherty, A. and Holtzman, D.M., Apolipoprotein E-containing high density lipoprotein promotes neurite outgrowth and is a ligand for the low density lipoprotein receptor-related protein, *J. Biol. Chem.*, 271 (1996) 30121-30125.

[12] Fujita, S.C., Sakuta, K., Tsuchiya, R. and Hamamaka, H., Apolipoprotein E is found in astrocytes but not in microglia in the normal mouse brain, *Neurosci. Res.*, 35 (1999) 123-133.

[13] Gong, J.-S., Kobayashi, M., Hayashi, H., Zou, K., Sawamura, N., Fujita, S.C., Yanagisawa, K. and Michikawa, M., Apolipoprotein E (ApoE) isoform-dependent lipid release from astrocytes prepared from human ApoE3 and ApoE4 knock in mice, *J. Biol. Chem.*, 277 (2002) 29919-29926.

[14] Hayashi, H., Campenot, R.B., Vance, D.E. and E., V.J., Apolipoprotein E-containing lipoproteins protect neurons from apoptosis via signaling pathway involving low-density lipoprotein receptor-related protein-1, *J. Neurosci.*, 27 (2007) 1933-1941.

[15] Hayashi, H., Campenot, R.B., Vance, D.E. and Vance, J.E., Glial lipoproteins stimulate axon growth of central nervous system neurons in compartmented cultures, *J. Biol. Chem.*, 279 (2004) 14009-14015.

[16] Hirsch-Reinshagen, V., Maia, L.F., Burgess, B.L., Blain, J.F., Naus, K.E., McIsaac, S.A., Parkinson, P.E., Chan, J.Y., Tansley, G.H. and Hayden, M.R., The absence of ABCA1 decreases soluble ApoE levels but does not diminish amyloid deposition in two murine models of Alzheimer disease, *J. Biol. Chem.*, 280 (2005) 43243-43256.

[17] Hirsch-Reinshagen, V., Zhou, S., Burgess, B.L., Bernier, L., Hayden, M.R. and Wellington, C.L., Deficiency of ABCA1 impairs apolipoprotein E metabolism in brain, *J. Biol. Chem.*, 279 (2004) 41197-41207.

[18] Hossain, W.A. and Morest, D.K., Fibroblast grwth factors (FGF-1, FGF-2) promote migration and neurite growth of mouse cocchlear ganglion cells in vitro: immunohistochemistry and antibody perturbation, *J. Neurosci. res.*, 62 (2000) 40-55.

[19] Ito, J.-i., Kheirollah, A., Nagayasu, Y., Lu, R., Kato, K. and Yokoyama, S., Apolipoprotein A-I increases association of cytosolic cholesterol and caveolin-1 with microtubule cytoskeletons in rat astrocytes., *J. Neurochem.*, 97 (2006) 1034-1043.

[20] Ito, J.-i., Li, H., Nagayasu, Y., Kheirollah, A. and Yokoyama, S., Apolipoprotein A-I induces translocation of protein kinase Calpha to a cytosolic lipid-protein particle in astrocytes, *J. Lipid Res.*, 45 (2004) 2269-2276.

[21] Ito, J.-i., Nagayasu, Y., Kato, K., sato, R. and Yokoyama, S., Apolipoprotein A-I induces translocation of cholesterol, phospholipid, and caveolin-1 to cytosol in rat astrocytes. *J. Biol. Chem., Vol. 277*, 2002a, pp. 7929-7935.

[22] Ito, J.-i., Nagayasu, Y., Kheirollah, A., Abe-Dohmae, S. and Yokoyama, S., ApoA-I enhances generation of HDL-like lipoproteins through interaction between ABCA1 and phospholipase Cgamma in rat strocytes, *Biochim. Biophys. Acta*, 1811 (2011) 1062-1069.

[23] Ito, J.-i., Nagayasu, Y., Lu, R., Kheirollah, A., Hayashi, M. and Yokoyama, S., Astrocytes produce and secrete FGF-1, which promotes the production of apoE-HDL in a manner of autocrine action, *J. Lipid Res.*, 46 (2005) 679-686.

[24] Ito, J.-i., Nagayasu, Y., Okumura-Noji, K., Lu, R., Nishida, T., Miura, Y., Asai, K., Kheirollah, A., Nakaya, S. and Yokoyama, S., Mechanism for FGF-1 to regulate biogenesis of apoE-HDL in astrocytes., *J. Lipid Res.*, 48 (2007) 2020-2027.

[25] Ito, J.-i., Nagayasu, Y., Ueno, S. and Yokoyama, S., Apolipoprotein-mediated cellular lipid release requires replenishment of sphingomyelin in a phosphatidylcholine-specific phospholipase C-dependent manner, *J. Biol. Chem.*, 277 (2002b) 44709-44714.

[26] Ito, J.-i., Zhang, L.-Y., Asai, M. and Yokoyama, S., Differential generation of high-density lipoprotein by endogenous and exogenous apolipoproteins in cultured fetal rat astrocytes, *J. Neurochem.*, 72 (1999) 2362-2369.

[27] Jackson, A., Friedman, S., Zhan, X., Engleka, K.A., Forough, R. and Maciag, T., Heat shock induces the release of fibroblast growth factor 1 from NIH3T3 cells, *Proc. Natl. Acad. Sci. U. S. A.*, 89 (1992) 10691-10695.

[28] Jiang, Q., Lee, C.Y., Mandrekr, S., Wilkinson, B., Cramer, P., Zelcer, N., mann, K., Lamb, B., Wilkinson, B., Cramer, P., Zelcer, N., Mann, K., Lamb, B., Willson, T.M. and Collins, J.L., ApoE promotes the proteolytic degradation of Abeta, *Neuron*, 58 (2008) 681-693.

[29] Kheirollah, A., Ito, J.-i., Nagayasu, Y., Lu, R. and Yokoyama, S., Cyclosporin A inhibits apolipoprotein A-I-induced early events in cellular cholesterol homeostasis in rat astrocytes., *Neuropharmacol.*, 51 (2006) 693-700.

[30] Koch, S., Donarski, N., Goetze, K., Kreckel, M., Stuerenburg, H.-J., Buhmann, C. and Beisiegel, U., Characterization of four lipoprotein classes in human cerebrospinal fluid, *J. Lipid. Res.*, 42 (2001) 1143-1151.

[31] Kockx, M., Guo, D.L., Huby, T., Lesnik, P., Kay, J., Sabarentnam, T., Jary, E., Hill, M., Gaus, K., Chapman, J., Stow, J.L., Jessup, W. and Kritharides, L., Secretion of apolipoprotein E from macrophages occurs via a protein kinase A-and calcium-dependent pathway along the microtubule network, *Circulation Res.*, 101 (2007) 607-616.

[32] Koldamova, R., Staufenbiel, M. and Lefterov, I., Lack of ABCA1 considerably decreases brain ApoE level and increases amyloid deposition in APP23 mice, *J. Biol. Chem.*, 280 (2005) 43224-43235.

[33] Larsson, H., Klint, P., Landgren, E. and Claesson-Welsh, L., Fibroblast growth factor receptor-1-mediated endothelial cell proliferation is dependent on the Src homology (SH)2/SH3 domain-containing adaptor protein Crk., *J. Biol. Chem.*, 274 (1999) 25726-25734.

[34] LaVallee, T.M., Tarantini, F., Gamble, S., Carreira, C.M., Jackson, A. and Maciag, T., Synaptotagmin-1 is required for fibroblast growth factor-1 release, *J. Biol. Chem.*, 273 (1998) 22217-22223.

[35] Lee, Y., Aono, M., Laskowitz, D., Warner, D.S. and Pearistein, R.D., Apolipoprotein E protects against oxidative stress in mixed neuronal-glial cell cultures by reducing glutamate toxicity, *Neurochem. Int.*, 44 (2004) 107-118.

[36] Linton, M.F., Gish, R., Hubl, S.T., Butler, E., Esquivel, C., Bry, W.L., Boyles, J.K., Wardell, M.R. and Young, S.G., Phenotypes of apolipoprotein B and E after liver transplantation., *J. Clin. Invest.*, 88 (1991) 270-281.

[37] Lu, R., Ito, J.-i., Iwamoto, N., Nishimaki-Mogami, T. and Yokoyama, S., FGF-1 induces expression of LXR and production of 25-hydroxycholesterol to upregulate the apoE gene in rat astrocytes, *J. Lipid Res.*, in press (2009).

[38] Mashayekhi, F., Hadavi, M., Vaziri, H.R. and Naji, M., Increased acidic fibroblast growth factor concentrations in the serum and cerebrospinal fluid of patients with Alzheimer's disease., *J. Clin. Neurosci.*, 17 (2010) 357-359.

[39] Mason, I.J., The ins and outs of fibroblast growth factors, *Cell*, 78 (1994) 547-552.

[40] Michikawa, M. and Yanagisawa, K., Apolipoprotein E4 induces neuronal cell death under conditions of suppressed de novo cholesterol synthesis., *J. Neurosci. Res.*, 54 (1998) 58-67.

[41] Minagawa, H., Gong, J.-S., Jung, C.G., Watanabe, A., Lund-Katz, S., Pillips, M.C., Saito, H. and Michikawa, M., Mechanism underlying apolipoprotein E (ApoE) isoform-dependent lipid efflux from neural cells in culture, *J. Neurosci. Res.*, 87 (2009) 2498-2508.

[42] Mockel, B., zinke, H., Flach, R., Weis, B., Weiler-Guttler, H. and gassen, H.G., Expression of apolipoprotein A-I in porcine brain endothelium in vitro, *J. Neurochem.*, 62 (1994) 788-798.

[43] Mulder, M., Ravid, R., Swaab, D.F., De Kloet, E.R., Haasdijk, E.D., Julk, J., Van Der Boom, J.J. and Havekes, L.M., Reduced levels of cholesterol, phospholipids, and fatty acids in cerebrospinal fluid of Alzheimer disease patients are not related to apolipoprotein E4., *Alzheimer Dis. Assoc. Disord.*, 12 (1998) 198-203.

[44] Nagayasu, Y., Ito, J.-i., Nishida, T. and Yokoyama, S., Reactivity of astrocytes to fibroblast growth factor-1 for biogenesis of apolipoprotein E-high density lipoprotein is down-regulated by long-time secondary culture, *J. Biochem. (Tokyo)*, 143 (2008) 611-616.

[45] Nakagawa, T. and Schwartz, J.P., Expression of neurotrophic factors and cytokines and their receptors on astrocytes in vivo, *Advances in Molecular and Cell Biology*, 31 (2004) 561-573.

[46] Nishida, T., Ito, J.-i., Nagayasu, Y. and yokoyama, S., FGF-1-induced reactions for biogenesis of apoE-HDL are mediated by Src in rat astrocytes, *J. Biochem.*, 146 (2009) 881-886.

[47] Ornitz, D.M., J. Xu, J.S., Colvin, D.G., McEwen, C.A., MacArthur, F., Coulier, G. and Gao, M.G., Receptor apecificity of the fibroblast growth factor family, *J. Biol. Chem.*, 271 (1996) 15292-15297.

[48] Snipes, G.J., McGuire, C.B., Norden, J.J. and Freeman, J.A., Nerve injury stimulates the secretion of apolipoprotein E by nonneuronal cells, *Proc. Natl. Acad. Sci. U. S. A.*, 83 (1986) 1130-1134.

[49] Tada, T., Ito, J.-i., Asai, M. and yokoyama, S., Fibroblast growth factor 1 is produced prior to apolipoprotein E in the astrocytes after cryo-injury of mouse brain, *Neurochem. Int.*, 45 (2004) 23-30.

[50] Takami, K., Matsuo, A., Terai, K., Walker, D.G., McGeer, E.G. and McGeer, P.L., Fibroblast growth factor receptor-1 expression in the eoctex and hippocampus in Alzheimer's Disease, *Brain Res.*, 802 (1998) 89-97.

[51] Thorns, V. and Masliah, E., Evidense for neuroprotective efffects of acidic fibroblast growth factor in Alzheimer disease., *J. Neuropathol. Exp. Neurol.*, 58 (1999) 296-306.

[52] Tooyama, I., Akiyama, H., McGeer, P.L., hara, Y., yasuhara, O. and Kimura, H., Acidic fibroblast growth factor-like immunoreactivity in brain of Alzheimer patients, *Neurosci. Lett.*, 121 (1991) 155-158.

[53] Ueno, S., Ito, J.-i., Nagayasu, Y., Furukawa, T. and Yokoyama, S., An acidic fibroblast growth factor-like factor secretedinto the brain cell culture medium upregulates apoE synthesis, HDL secretion and cholesterol metabolism in rat astrocytes, *Biochim. Biophys. Acta*, 1589 (2002) 261-272.

[54] Wahrle, S.E., Jiang, H., Parsadanian, M., Hartman, R.E., Bales, K.R., Paul, S.M. and Holzman, D.M., Deletion of Abca1 increases Abeta deposition in the PDAPP transgenic mouse model of Alzheimer Disease, *J. Biol. Chem.*, 280 (2005) 43236-43242.

[55] Wahrle, S.E., Jiang, H., Parsadanian, M., Kim, J., Li, A., Knoten, A., Jain, S., Hirsch-Reinshagen, V., Wellington, C.L. and Bales, K.R., Overexpression of ABCA1 reduces amyloid deposition in the PDAPP mouse model of Alzheimer disease, *J. Clin. Invest.*, 118 (2008) 671-682.

[56] Wahrle, S.E., Jiang, H., Parsadanian, M., Legleiter, J., Han, X., Fryer, J.D., Kowalewski, T. and Holtzman, D.M., ABCA1 is required for normal central nervous system apoE levels and for lipidation of astrocytes-secreted apoE, *J. Biol. Chem.*, 279 (2004) 40987-40993.

[57] Wiedlocha, A., Nilsen, T., Wesche, J., Sorensen, V., Malecki, J., Marcinkowska, E. and Olsnes, S., Phosphorylation-regulated nucleocytoplasmic trafficking of internalized fibroblast growth factor-1, *Mol. Biol. Cell*, 16 (2005) 794-810.

[58] Zannis, V.I., McPherson, J., Goldberger, G., Karathanasis, S. and Breslow, j.L., Synthesis, intracellular processing, and signal peptide of human apolipoprotein E, *J. Biol. Chem.*, 259 (1984) 5495-5499.

[59] Zhao, Y. and Mazzone, T., Transport and processing of endogenously synthesized apoE on the macrophage cell surface, *J. Biol. Chem.*, 275 (2000) 4759-4765.

Index

G

H

I

K

L

M

N